END

ENDING PAIN

Coaching the Body with Neuroscience, Movement and Trigger Point Therapy

CHUCK DUFF

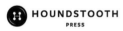

HOUNDSTOOTH
PRESS

Hardcover ISBN: 978-1-5445-3336-0
Paperback ISBN: 978-1-5445-3337-7
Ebook ISBN: 978-1-5445-3338-4

CONTENTS

INTRODUCTION

Why I Wrote This Book

I know what it feels like to hurt so badly you can't get off the floor. As a bodyworker, I've observed not only the pervasiveness of chronic pain but also how much it is misunderstood and misdiagnosed. Our medical system's deep misunderstanding of pain is literally killing us, causing financial despair, depression, anxiety, lost careers, and compromised enjoyment of life. Traditional medicine also enables a culture of uninformed dependency that is both damaging and unnecessary.

I know there is another way, a different and more lasting solution for common pain complaints such as back pain, shoulder pain, and sciatica. The approach I've developed doesn't require addictive prescription opioids, exotic medical equipment, or billions of dollars in research.

The system I will present to you in this book has been tested for many years over thousands of clinical sessions performed by my students and myself, and I know it works. Patient outcome is the only criterion I care about. I'm a practical person, and I don't argue the merits of an academic approach without the test of experience. I put ideas into practice, assess them honestly, and keep what works.

What I've discovered is that resolving pain isn't even that difficult—but it does require open-mindedness and a willingness to see things in a new way. Pain relief "only" requires us to reset what we believe about what causes pain and a thorough analysis of how the body's compensations cause common pain patterns. I say "only" because I do not underestimate the difficulty of changing or undoing age-old beliefs about pain that are conveniently supported by corporate profit motives. But if you're willing to give these ideas and methods a try, effective pain relief is within your reach.

Despite how many practitioners struggle to successfully treat pain in any kind of lasting way, it's not rocket science. What you can learn in this book is an efficient, remarkably fast, and effective system for removing extremely common, hidden sources of muscular disturbance known by a select few as "myofascial trigger points."

Briefly, trigger points in muscles generate "danger signals" that are sent to the central nervous system. The central nervous system (CNS) evaluates the stream of danger signals to assess the threat level, and based on that assessment, the brain may choose to "output" what we know and feel as pain. My system involves hacking the CNS by offering it an experience of movement without pain, giving the CNS "evidence-based reasons" to drop its hyper-protective stance that caused the pain in the first place.

Trigger point therapy was formulated by MDs Janet Travell and David Simons in their two-volume seminal book, *The Trigger Point Manual.* These medical textbooks were the result of a brilliant, monumental effort, but the trigger point approach has failed to gain wide acceptance outside of a tiny minority of practitioners. In this book, I address the reasons why I believe that trigger point therapy has largely been marginalized. I will present some additions based on modern neuroscience, a new method of analysis, and manual therapy techniques that I have found to produce dramatic results. Since its original formulation in 2005, my Coaching the

Body method has proven to be a reliable and consistent approach for treating pain at its true source, even in cases that have eluded many other practitioners.

Who This Book Is For

While the principles behind my system are based in anatomy and neuroscience, they are accessible to any curious individual willing to learn. Although medical language can be daunting, I've taught many students successfully who had no prior experience in the field. I see my audience for this book as three general groups: professionals who are familiar with anatomy and wish to increase success with their clients; movement and exercise instructors who are less familiar with anatomy but would like to help their clients; and interested individuals who are willing to learn some medical language in the service of self-care or helping a loved one.

I know from many years of teaching this system to people from all walks of life that anyone can learn the necessary concepts and language. Regardless of who you are—massage therapist, yoga or movement instructor, personal trainer, health coach, psychotherapist, physical therapist, medical doctor, athlete, dancer, or an enthusiastic non-professional—you will gain some important ideas and techniques from this book. I want to put my system in your hands and empower you with knowledge to help yourself and others. In this way, we can change our deeply flawed pain industry from the ground up, one improved life at a time.

This Is What You Can Expect to Learn

Most of us don't understand pain, but we all experience it. The Western medical system generally sees pain as a sign of something broken that needs fixing—as a manifestation of injury or disease, an inevitable consequence of damaged tissues. This pathology model of pain is both thoroughly inculcated into popular thinking and, unfortunately, wrong in most cases. Even when medical imaging shows departures from the "normal" in body tissues, the widespread assumption that those findings are the cause of pain denies the insights of modern neuroscience and leads to ineffective treatments, unnecessary interventions, and disturbed—even ruined—lives.

My goals for you are myriad: to help you find a new way of understanding pain so that you might be motivated to learn more and become as successful as we are at lasting healing, to impart some practical techniques that you can try on yourself or your associates, and to provide some encouragement that it's appropriate to question the misguided medical assumptions that have failed many patients. My ultimate goal is to foster change within a system that imposes unnecessary suffering upon untold millions each year via inappropriate, ineffective, and invasive procedures and medications by offering a safe and legal alternative to opioids and surgery.

While these pages contain many practical examples and demonstrations, I intentionally have not written this book as a how-to manual. Complete coverage of my Coaching the Body system would take far more than a single book. However, I believe that this material will give you a useful and significant first step on your way to understanding a unique and new way of approaching pain that includes both analysis and technique.

If you wish to go deeper, we offer many helpful resources. You will find many examples in the book, along with accompanying videos that you can view on our website via links and QR codes. I prefer to do my demonstrations, whenever possible, on people who have real and relevant pain issues so that you, as the viewer, can see my decision-making in action and also see the actual, patient-specific results.

A Guide to the Chapter Contents

In 2001, I embarked upon a quest to discover a better way to treat pain in my clients and myself. My work in creating Coaching the Body (CTB) came out of the fabric of my own life, including a serious recurring pain issue that is now fully resolved using CTB principles and practices. In Chapter 1, you will get to know some of my history and what led to my encounter with Thai massage and trigger point therapy. I had studied traditional Thai massage as a means of helping people but found my results from traditional techniques to be erratic and short-lived. As I worked with more clients, I was shocked at how most of them had been failed by both traditional medical and alternative approaches. I came across the field of trigger point therapy during that time and was immediately fascinated. But as I investigated further, I encountered some issues that limited its adoption, some missing pieces, and a spotty track record with therapists who mostly weren't well trained. I had an intuitive sense that my work was on the right track, and thankfully I persisted.

In Chapter 2, I'll discuss the dimensions of the ongoing pain crisis that ruins lives, causes financial despair, and even kills people. In 2020 alone, amidst a worldwide pandemic, 100,000 people died due to opioid overdose, exacerbating an existing trend that has spanned many years. These terrible statistics derive directly from a misunderstanding of the origins of pain along with corporate greed. Most of the medical system ignores the insights of trigger point therapy and neuroscience—instead, ascribing the origins of pain to injury, which is far more profitable.

Chapter 3 goes into more depth about the history of pain theories and exciting recent developments in neuroscience that inform the principles behind Coaching the Body. I'll discuss how these insights, together with trigger point theory, provided a starting point for my approach.

In order to understand CTB, it's necessary to understand trigger point principles. In Chapter 4, I summarize trigger point theory along with some new ideas that begin to integrate the work of Travell and Simons with my approach to pain.

When muscles develop trigger points, they can misbehave in a variety of ways that confuse medical practitioners, who assume an injury at the site of the pain. Chapter 5 goes into detail about the surprising ways that trigger points can disrupt muscular function and masquerade as more serious conditions.

Chapter 6 explores the reasons why trigger point therapy has never achieved wide acceptance, and I present some modifications and additions to the approach that make it much more reliably effective. The chapter concludes with several practical examples. I demonstrate in concrete terms the importance of satellite referral and muscle function in getting to the true source of pain.

In Chapter 7, I summarize the principles of Coaching the Body. These principles guide our approach and present a new understanding of how trigger points in peripheral muscles confuse the overprotective central nervous system, which leads to chronic pain. We cannot get to the root of a pain condition without understanding muscle networks and how they collaborate to cause pain. These principles guide every aspect of our therapy. I present a more effective method of analysis that integrates functional relationships and satellite referral.

In Chapter 8, I present our core protocols for upper and lower body pain complaints that guide practitioners in treating the appropriate network of muscles in the proper sequence. This effort must take into account the hidden relationships that are the key to effective, lasting treatment. Protocols are the key to designing effective treatments in a reasonable amount of time and are one of the most valuable contributions of the CTB system.

Chapter 9 describes the CTB treatment cycle. A protocol consists of a flexible and tunable series of treatments for the muscles most likely contributing to pain conditions in the upper or lower body. Within each muscle treatment, practitioners are guided by the CTB treatment cycle, which establishes a general formula for resolving trigger points in muscles. Specific muscles may depart somewhat from the general, but it is an excellent model that provides a guide for effective treatment of trigger points.

Each muscle has its own treatment characteristics. In Chapter 10, I go into depth on a sampling of the techniques we have developed, focusing on the muscles that they target and the rationale guiding each technique's specific features. In the CTB system, techniques are secondary to accurate analysis, but we've developed an extensive repertoire of excellent, effective techniques for each muscle. Many of our techniques have emerged from Thai massage but are modified by the deep muscle knowledge contained in the CTB system.

CTB is known for its use of therapeutic vibration, with such tools as the Muscle Liberator. Chapter 11 discusses the science that motivates our use of therapeutic vibration, as well as our use of the electronic point stimulator (EPS). We take a radically different approach to vibration and electronic stimulation, one that supports our overall goals and treatment cycle.

The CTB principles and treatment cycle can be applied to self-care techniques in the same manner as we've designed our manual therapy techniques. For therapists who are unlicensed or uncomfortable with hands-on therapy, self-care techniques can be a valuable asset for helping their clients. In Chapter 12, I present a sampling of our self-care techniques for major muscles, along with guidelines for extending this self-treatment model to other muscles.

Ultimately, trigger points develop as a response to overload, imbalance, or instability in the body, set up by perpetuating factors that we have found to be present in a majority of cases. Chapter

13 discusses the most important of these perpetuating factors, including leg length discrepancy, hyperpronation, breathing dysfunction, and more.

CTB is not just for bodyworkers. Chapter 14 discusses the application of CTB principles to other movement arts, such as personal training, yoga, and Pilates. Using our refined approach to analysis and an understanding of the effects of movements on muscles, non-bodyworkers can add a powerful dimension to their offerings.

Finally, in Chapter 15, I offer some additional online resources for readers who desire more in-depth knowledge about our CTB approach to pain treatment.

CHAPTER 1

My Path to Pain-Free

Creating the Coaching the Body approach, investigating the true sources of pain in the body, and helping countless people find relief has been a winding and sometimes frustrating path. While today I am pain-free and focused on helping others, my interest in treating pain began with my own serious pain issues and the total failure of the doctors and therapists I visited to adequately treat them.

Beginning in my teenage years, I would experience bouts of severe, disabling pain, primarily in my low back and hips. Being an athletic young man, I didn't take it very seriously, and as athletes, we were taught that pain is just part of the lifestyle.

When I became a bodyworker, I began to realize that pain is almost universal. Most of my clients were seeking relief for their chronic or acute pain, having been failed or dismissed by medical doctors and other professionals.

It doesn't have to be this way. There is a solution, but it took me years of curiosity, investigation, and experimentation—not to mention client and student trust—to find it.

The Case of the Disappearing "Heel Spur"

When I was in high school, I ran track. The long jump, one of my events, involves running as fast as you can and launching off a board at the end of the track. Your forward momentum propels you into the air, launched by an explosive effort from the calf muscles when the ball of your foot pushes off the board.

Eventually, I developed heel pain so severe that I couldn't compete. My family doctor diagnosed me with a heel spur, a calcified outgrowth on the bottom of my calcaneus, or heel bone. He didn't even order an X-ray; he just recommended getting a padded heel cup.

Even then, I found the diagnosis questionable. First of all, my heel didn't hurt to the touch, only when I walked. Secondly, I thought it was strange that my body would just randomly develop a spur like that. My events and style of running focused on the ball of the foot, not the heel, so I wasn't pounding my heel constantly. In addition, wearing the padded cup didn't relieve or eliminate the pain. It just didn't add up.

Regardless, I stopped long jumping, and eventually, the pain disappeared. I concluded, with some degree of suspicion, that the "heel spur" had magically dissolved. But I knew something was amiss. Even so, I had to stop doing a sport I enjoyed because my doctor didn't have the tools or knowledge to treat my pain.

Harnessing the Power of Opposites

I've had success throughout my life by combining seemingly very different approaches to seed the creation of something new. That has certainly been the case with Coaching the Body.

I was a very rational child. It's only fitting that I was a science nerd, and my family was convinced that I would become a doctor. One of my most memorable and exciting Christmas gifts was a visual model of the human head.

I also loved discovering how things worked. In high school, I would tear apart my cars and electronic equipment. I'd spend hours reading my parents' *Encyclopedia Britannica* from the 1930s, poring over the development of aviation, Marie Curie's discoveries, and the precursors of modern science. At the same time, I loved art and music; I drew, painted, and studied piano and guitar. I knew that I had feelings, but I had few tools for expressing or processing them, and it was easier to just ignore them, more or less. Even then, my life seemed to be defined by the power of opposites.

After high school, I entered the University of Chicago in 1971, planning to major in physics, and soon was exposed to all manner of fascinating people. Inspired by the beat poets, I began reading about Buddhism, doing LSD, and discovering an entire universe that I didn't even know existed.

But the healing power of psychedelics couldn't prevent more serious pain from showing up in my body. In addition to my heel pain, my continued guitar practice brought with it forearm and wrist pain; both were primarily from overuse. I started to experience a more severe, sometimes crippling, recurring pain pattern in my low back. Doctors prescribed me a muscle relaxer and rest. The pain would fade, but it interested me because I had no idea why it was happening. My drive to understand things led me on a winding and fortuitous journey.

Early in my freshman year, I enrolled in an intriguingly titled course, *Thoughts and Feelings,* taught by Eugene Gendlin, and my life was forever changed. Gendlin was a psychologist and philosopher who studied with the great psychologist Carl Rogers at the University of Chicago. He's best known for two formal processes he called Focusing and Listening. In his class, he used Socratic dialogue as a means of discovering a higher level of truth via dialogue between principles that are separate and, in some ways, even opposed—in this case, thoughts and feelings. I had never had any kind of structured opportunity to discuss my feelings before, let alone in a classroom at the intellectual bastion of the University of Chicago under a great philosopher's tutelage.

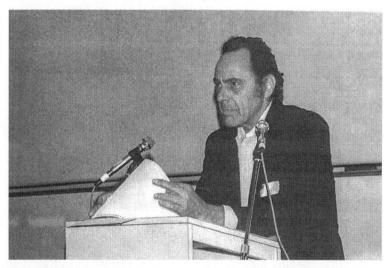

Fig. 1-1. The American philosopher, Eugene Gendlin. Credit: Aparna Sandeep at English Wikipedia, under Creative Commons Attribution-Share Alike 4.0 International.

In retrospect, I can see how Gendlin's dialectic model has been a pervasive influence in my life. The idea of exploring the tension in a dyad of opposites, allowing a new, original solution to emerge, has proven a powerful formula that I have usefully pursued a few times over.

At the end of my freshman year, I had an internal sea change and made a dramatic shift away from my science path. I became the first student in a new, integrative program of study: Religion and the Humanities. Following the dialectic idea, I was very interested in exploring the relationship between psychotherapy and Buddhist philosophy, focused primarily on a comparative study of Sigmund Freud and Carl Jung.

After graduating, I studied for a summer at the newly founded Naropa Institute in Boulder, Colorado, where the Tibetan master Chögyam Trungpa Rinpoche was assembling a world-class community of thinkers, artists, poets, musicians, and hippie seekers like me. I constantly had to remind myself that it wasn't a dream.

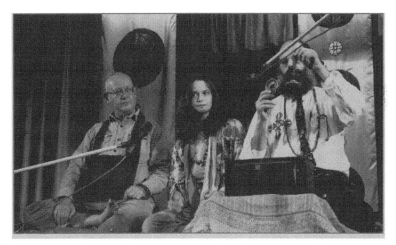

Fig. 1-2. Philip Whalen, Anne Waldman, and Alan Ginsberg giving a reading at Naropa Institute, 1975. Photograph by Rachel Homer.

I studied music alongside luminaries like Robben Ford, who toured with Joni Mitchell as her guitarist and arranger, and attended lectures with monumental thinkers like Gregory Bateson. I also found myself in a small poetry class taught by one of my beat heroes, Alan Ginsberg, who would read our journals and recite his favorite passages from one of his own mentors, William Carlos Williams. It was an amazing, intoxicating opportunity for a curious young man trying to find his way.

It seemed, though, that my path would not be linear. Life's necessities took over, and I needed to work and get a job. I didn't have any financial cushion, and my mother was getting on in years, so I eventually returned to Chicago, where I worked as a bartender and went to chef school.

While working as a chef, I attended classes in computer science at the University of Illinois Chicago Circle (UIC) and began a master's degree. My background in physics and my natural creativity made me uniquely suited for the now exploding world of personal computing. I studied with Thomas DeFanti, a prodigy who became a full professor at eighteen; his lab generated the 3D graphics for the trench scene in the first Star Wars film.

After spending a few years at UIC, I grew tired of academics and eventually found my calling in designing programming languages for brand new PC platforms. I again applied the dialectic concept I learned from Gendlin in combining two concurrent trends.

I integrated some newly emerging object-oriented programming ideas, best represented in a language called Smalltalk, developed by Xerox PARC research group, with a very minimal, esoteric language called FORTH that Charles Moore had developed to control radio telescopes. I created NEON, a new language that combined the best of these approaches and became the first interactive, object-oriented language for the Macintosh. NEON was later used by Dr. Robert Lowenstein, an infrared astronomer, as a control system on a Space Shuttle mission. I subsequently applied my learnings from that first project and created Actor, the first interactive programming language for Windows 1.0.

But several changes made it clear that I didn't want to stay in computing for much longer. What had first been a field full of creativity and exploration became commodified and taken over by big business interests.

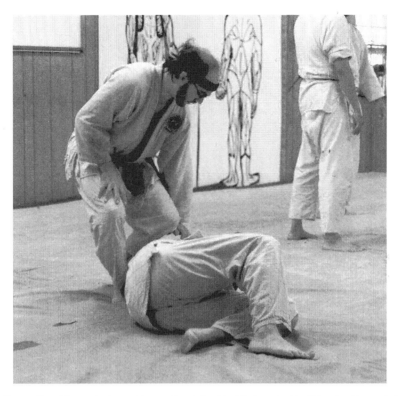

Fig. 1-3. Practicing a takedown with one of my fellow black belts at the Hapkido school I attended for twelve years under Master Kwang Seek Hyun. The efficiency and circular movement patterns of Hapkido have powerfully informed my approach to body mechanics. Credit: Vic Cushing.

In addition, my many years of sitting—as well as the stress of a fast-paced and growing industry—had started to take their toll on my body. Even though I was in very good shape, the many hours sitting in front of computers combined with twelve years of vigorous Hapkido workouts—where I hit the floor repeatedly while practicing takedowns—had taken my lower back pain from bad to worse. While a yoga practice helped, the pain was disabling on a regular basis.

After starting several software companies, raising venture capital, and having a couple of them acquired, I felt that I had the financial means to do something more explicitly helpful to people, not to mention kinder to my own body and spirit. I accepted my natural desire to understand and began exploring more therapeutic movement modalities.

I would take my lunch break at the tech company where I served as Chief Technical Officer and began going to a local bookstore, just pulling books off the shelf and seeing what ideas and possibilities arose in me. I did that for close to a year before I began to settle on Thai massage. As I look back, I was guided in some manner toward this path, even though my thinking was still confused as to what would be best.

Journeying into Thai Massage

In the late 1990s, in an effort to ease my beaten down body and soul, I began traveling to the Harbin Hot Springs spa in the Northern California high desert, where I'd receive Thai massage sessions. Thai massage, with its yoga-like emphasis on movement and stretches, seemed like a logical and intuitive way to address my own pain. It worked well enough that I decided to learn how to practice it myself, first as a way to keep some movement in my life and then to hopefully help some people as I continued my software career. I studied in the United States, Thailand, and Canada, and I began practicing part-time.

Little did I know at the time that taking this step would lead me to my next great adventure.

One of my instructors encouraged me to teach, and before very long, I had a growing class schedule with students coming to learn from all over. While I hadn't initially intended to pursue this path full-time, it seemed that the energy was there, and the students and clients were showing up. I found myself revisiting Buddhism and healing in a very interesting way that I hadn't done since college. Fortunately, in a relatively short time, we were able to build Thai Bodywork School into a national presence.

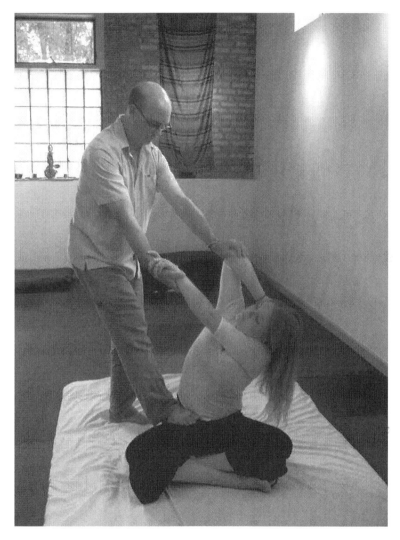

Fig. 1-5. Showing a Thai spinal twist in 2006 with my daughter, Rachel, who has studied with me since age sixteen and is now a photographer, dancer, and CTB practitioner based in Oakland, CA.

At first, I didn't exclusively focus on helping people with pain. I had just hoped to learn something that could keep people healthy and relieve stress and would enable me to lead a more active lifestyle. However, the universe had other things in store for me.

As my own practice grew in the early 2000s, I began attracting many people who were experiencing various kinds of pain. My awareness grew that beyond my own issues, chronic pain was a widespread and poorly understood problem.

In the beginning, this was a bit frightening and overwhelming. I had learned a lot of fancy tricks and techniques, but not how to apply them to specific pain conditions. Traditional Thai training includes little or no study of musculoskeletal anatomy, but clients were coming to me with shoulder pain, low back pain, sciatica, foot pain, headaches, and pretty much everything imaginable. Most of them had been done a disservice by the practitioners they had seen, medical and otherwise. I wanted to help them, not become one more disappointment.

I knew that I needed additional tools. I began to see a new opportunity for applying Gendlin's process of dialectic in the form of a dialogue between the traditional bodywork approach of Thai massage and a relatively obscure offshoot of Western medicine called trigger point therapy.

Discovering Trigger Point Therapy

In 2001, I discovered Clair Davies's *Trigger Point Workbook*, and I made a fascinating connection between the heel pain I had in high school and the Thai bodywork I'd been practicing. As I read through the chapter about the soleus—a powerful calf muscle that supplies most of the propulsion required for the long jump—I was shocked to find a description of the exact pain pattern from my high school days. The soleus can cause pain in the Achilles tendon and the heel all by itself—no bone spurs, arthritis, or injuries required.

Things started to make sense. My track events required short, explosive, and powerful engagement of the soleus. When I stopped competing and using the muscles in that way, my pain subsided. In addition, Davies points out that many medical doctors (I'd say most of them) who diagnose heel pain as a "bone spur" know little to nothing about trigger points.

I sought out and studied with Clair Davies, which led to my intensive study of the medical textbooks that defined the trigger point therapy field, such as Travell and Simons's definitive two-volume publication, *Myofascial Pain and Dysfunction*. And they confirmed my high school suspicion that our family doctor had missed an important source of my pain: the muscles. In fact, Travell

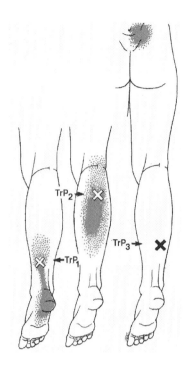

Fig. 1-6. Heel pain is one of the most common pain referral patterns of the soleus muscle.

and Simons cite a number of studies that show that *muscles cause the majority of pain, both chronic and acute.*[1]

This heel pain scenario from my own life perfectly illustrates a ubiquitous problem with the medical profession's understanding of pain. I call it "injury-centric thinking," as in trying to find *the injury or disease at the site of the pain*, such as a tear, a break, arthritis, bursitis, or impingement of a nerve at the spine due to disk compression. Medical doctors hardly consider muscle dysfunction as a possible pain source unless some kind of tear is involved.

---

1   Janet G. Travell and David G. Simons, *Myofascial Pain and Dysfunction, Vol. 1: The Trigger Point Manual, The Upper Extremities* (Baltimore: Williams & Wilkins, 1982), 30–32.

Here was an opportunity for me to address the pain in so many of the people seeking out my approach to bodywork. Treat the muscles and relieve the pain.

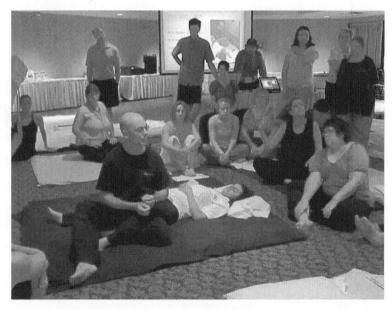

Fig. 1-7. Presenting a workshop at the National Association of Myofascial Trigger Point Therapists conference in 2010.

Integrating Trigger Point Therapy into Thai Massage

I began experimenting with Thai techniques as a vehicle to implement trigger point principles. Along the way, I found that in spite of the profound breakthroughs in trigger point theory, its practical application in manual therapy was very limited due to its medical origins.

The original books on trigger point therapy had been written by and for doctors, and the preferred treatment method was injection of a local anesthetic, procaine hydrochloride. They included virtually no coverage of manual therapy. As a result, Travell and Simons's work had found very limited acceptance in the manual therapy field. In addition, very few doctors were willing to take on this complex practice, given the limitations of covering their time via medical billing and the fact that very few general practitioners have the kind of thorough understanding of muscular anatomy that trigger point therapy requires.

I knew that I needed to fully understand the muscular effects of the Thai technique repertoire because trigger point work is focused on normalizing muscles. Because I had learned little or no anatomy in my traditional studies, I began intense study of kinesiology and functional anatomy. I learned any time a joint moves, it shortens some muscles and stretches others. With that knowledge, I dissected the Thai techniques, pose by pose, analyzing the way each affects the muscles and their corresponding joints.

As I studied the true effects of hundreds of Thai poses, I was also learning the trigger point characteristics of each muscle. I went through a long process of modifying the Thai techniques to be more useful treatments for specific muscles, and I began experimenting with point stimulator devices that I had encountered while on staff at Pacific College of Oriental Medicine. I found the Travell spray and stretch drawings to be very helpful in developing range of motion techniques for each muscle. Using my own body and my clients as subjects, I was developing a new approach to treating pain. Even then, my efforts were at least partially successful, and my clients didn't complain about my experiments. Most were eager to experience my new tricks and discoveries each week.

Once I started applying the Thai techniques supported by my growing knowledge of trigger points, I could see the synergistic power of this combination. I began to experience success in most of my sessions. I used these same ideas on myself, and through my evolving version of trigger point treatment (and a new approach to my yoga practice, which focused on Ashtanga), I eliminated my own severe low back pain that had nagged me for so long.

Creating Coaching the Body

Even though I had already opened a school to teach Thai massage, my students were eager to learn more about my incorporation of trigger points. I wanted to teach them, but I knew I had to become more proficient at employing these ideas and having a more fully developed theoretical framework before I tried teaching it to others.

My years of Thai massage training had been based primarily upon imitation. And while I could rely on my strong intuition as a practitioner—using certain tricks I knew were effective without full certainty why they worked—I was frustrated that my teachers never explained the justification, analysis, or understanding of why a given technique was appropriate. I vowed when I became a teacher never to do that to my students. As a teacher, I felt strongly that I needed to be able to explain *why* methods worked. With my newfound success, I felt a lot of pressure, both self-generated and external, to get my work into the world.

At the same time, more and more people in the United States were turning to prescription drugs to address their chronic pain, including the highly addictive OxyContin. If I could offer a drug-free approach to pain relief, then I needed to make sure the method was as complete as possible.

I spent many years putting together protocols that identified the most important muscles for each pain complaint, the best order of treatment, appropriate techniques, and how to make decisions about altering treatment order and skipping sections based on continual assessment during treatment. I'll go into much more detail on our protocols later in the book.

In 2005, I taught my first workshop covering what I called Clinical Thai Bodywork, which I later changed to Coaching the Body (CTB) because it had evolved considerably away from the Thai massage framework.

Why I Want You to Read This Book

In my career, I have observed the pervasiveness of widespread pain, the harm it does to your well-being, and the reliance on prescription drugs to mitigate the lasting effects. I have tested my approach over thousands of sessions and many years of research. If you follow my teachings with an open mind, you can begin to alleviate the pain without the use of expensive equipment or addictive opioids.

Because trigger point therapy has been severely limited in its success and professional acceptance, I'm proposing an update: Trigger Point 2.0. In this book, I'll cover:

- Modern ideas of neuroscience that offer a deeper understanding of the why behind pain, trigger point development, and muscle dysfunction, along with more effective treatment, coaching, and self-care strategies.

- Viable manual therapy techniques replacing static compression and injection with a more dynamic and integrative approach, including movement with feedback, therapeutic vibration, and electronic pulse stimulation while emphasizing neurological distraction.

- Replacing the single-muscle, direct referral analysis of the origins of pain with an emphasis on networks of muscles related by function, satellite referral, and neurological connections and a rational understanding of how these chains typically develop dysfunction.

This book will show you an efficient and effective system for removing extremely common, hidden sources of peripheral danger signals while "hacking" the CNS to decrease the cause of the pain. This sounds technical, but with an open mind and natural curiosity, you will gain a great understanding of the body from this book. My goal is to empower you with knowledge, and change the system from the ground up, one improved life at a time.

"My first personal experience with the true power of the CTB modality came only days after my first class focused on trigger point treatment. The course was on the shoulder, and I was determined to try my new techniques on my neighbor and dear friend—a woman in her sixties who had been on disability due to pain and dysfunction in her right should for the past fifteen years. Her pain had gotten worse over the previous couple of months, and the evening I decided to work on her, she told me she hadn't been able to lift her arm high enough to brush her teeth that morning. I knew I had my work cut out for me. I took my time, going through each portion of Chuck's shoulder protocol meticulously. The session took me a full three hours. When I had completed the protocol to the best of my ability, I had my friend sit up and try to lift her arm. We were both astounded when she lifted her arm clear over her head without pain. 'I haven't done this in years!' she exclaimed. I was overjoyed. Needless to say, she has come back to me many times over the past five years for her other shoulder, her knees, and her back. And luckily, my sessions no longer require three hours of her time."

—Zoë Verdin, CTB Advanced Practitioner
and CTBI School Administrator

CHAPTER 2

Our Pain Crisis

Chances are, you or someone you know suffers from chronic pain. Countless people throughout the United States go about their lives with persistent, troubling levels of pain. In recent years, not coincidentally, prime time television has become dominated by drug ads promising quick relief. In this chapter, I will survey the dimensions of the crisis and introduce some ideas that I believe represent a solution.

For the last several years, I've been advertising my teaching programs to practitioners on social media. I've been quite surprised by how many non-practitioners comment, ask questions, and even attend my practitioner webinars because they are in severe pain and haven't been able to find help. I would guess that for every practitioner interested in our material, we are contacted by five to ten non-professional people who are themselves in pain. People go to almost any length to find help for their pain because the medical system is largely failing them. To help that community benefit from our insights, we've created online courses on self-care for upper and lower body pain. These have seen a tremendous amount of demand.

Pain: A Brief Primer

In the next chapter, I will explain how pain is *not* a physical phenomenon determined by injury. The experience of pain is an output generated by the brain based on an assessment of many inputs, including emotional distress. Consequently, victimization and disempowerment are just as potent a perpetrator of pain as tissue damage and, in some ways, is much more so.

The body is very good at repairing damaged tissues in mere weeks, after which engaging with soft tissue is no longer fruitful for stopping pain. Chronic pain is almost never about injury; it is much more about the elevated state of vigilance and alertness that develops following a traumatic event. Unfortunately, the manner in which pain manifests, appearing in and near joints and other structures, tricks otherwise intelligent practitioners into assuming a local injury.

The central nervous system (CNS) works to maximize self-preservation in the face of danger, even if the danger is an illusion. Pain is part of this protective effort. Think of pain as analogous to the annoying screech from a smoke alarm, which alerts us to a possible problem (smoke). The smoke might, in fact, be coming from a cooking adventure and not a house fire. Trigger points are like high-heat cooking: they produce an impressive amount of smoke, but there's no real danger. All we need to do is vent the smoke and turn down the flame; no need for firefighters to come in and destroy the house.

Quantifying the Pain Epidemic

According to a study by the CDC in 2019, 20.4 percent of US adults experience significant chronic pain, meaning most or every day of their lives.[2] Other studies estimate instances of chronic pain

---

2   Carla E. Zelaya, et al., "Chronic Pain and High-impact Chronic Pain Among US Adults, 2019," Centers for Disease Control and Prevention NCHS Data Brief, no. 390, November 2020, https://www.cdc.gov/nchs/products/databriefs/db390.htm.

to be much higher, at 20–40 percent, with considerable variation between sub-populations. Age makes things worse: 65 percent of adults sixty-five and older report chronic pain. Of course, in any study like these, accuracy is limited by the level of reporting, and chronic pain is notoriously underreported.

Figure 1. National Drug-Involved Overdose Deaths*
Number Among All Ages, by Gender, 1999-2019

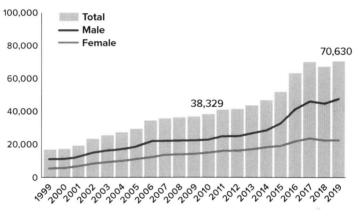

*Includes deaths with underlying causes of unintentional drug poisoning (X40-X44), suicide drug poisoning (X60-X64), homicide drug poisoning (X85), or drug poisoning of undetermined intent (Y10-Y14), as coded in the International Classification of Diseases, 10th Revision. Source: Centers for Disease Control and Prevention, National Center for Health Statistics. Multiple Cause of Death 1999-2019 on CDC WONDER Online Database, released 12/2020.

Fig. 2-1.

Chronic pain can lead to severe mental health consequences, too. Those reporting chronic pain are three times more likely to be diagnosed with depression and anxiety and are at twice the risk of suicide.

Many people turn to medications to treat their chronic pain, both at the recommendation of their doctor and because of increased marketing by pharmaceutical companies. According to a study by Georgetown University, 66 percent of all adults in the United States use prescription drugs, increasing with age. Of adults aged 40–79, 69.0 percent reported using one or more prescription drugs in the past thirty days, and 22.4 percent used five or more.[3] Many of these prescriptions are for painkillers; doctors write 259 million prescriptions for painkillers each year.

A significant portion of their painkillers are opioids, which are highly addictive, even when used as directed. In 2017, healthcare providers across the US wrote more than 191 million prescriptions for opioid pain medication—or 58.7 prescriptions per 100 people.[4] Indeed, opioid use skyrocketed after 1995, when Purdue Pharma began aggressively marketing OxyContin. OxyContin contains oxycodone—a very dangerous and addictive opioid—in a time-release form. Purdue Pharma ignored public health implications and created a new generation of addicts who sometimes transitioned to recreational abuse.[5] In fact, the National Institute on Drug Abuse found in 2019 that more than 80 percent of heroin users began with a legal prescription for opioids.[6] Approximately 21–29 percent of patients misuse prescription opioids, leading to 17,000 overdose deaths annually. Even so, people who use opioids for chronic pain are often unsatisfied; a survey by *Healthline* in 2018 found that medication only resolved pain for 5 percent of respondents. Moreover, 45 percent of respondents said that medication "wasn't enough" or "didn't help at all."[7] I consider the

---

3   "Prescription Drugs," Georgetown University Health Policy Institute, accessed August 5, 2021, https://hpi.georgetown.edu/rxdrugs.

4   "7 Staggering Statistics About America's Opioid Epidemic," Choose PT, May 9, 2016, https://www.choosept.com/resources/detail/7-staggering-statistics-about-america-s-opioid-epi.

5   For an in-depth investigation of the opioid crisis in the United States, I highly recommend watching *The Crime of the Century*, an HBO documentary.

6   "Opioid Overdose Crisis." National Institute on Drug Abuse, accessed August 10, 2021, https://www.drugabuse.gov/drugs-abuse/opioids/opioid-overdose-crisis.

7   Anna Wahrman and Whitney Akers, "America is Losing the War on Chronic Pain," *Healthline*, September 24, 2018, https://www.healthline.com/health-news/america-is-losing-the-war-on-chronic-pain.

opioid addiction and overdose crisis to be a direct manifestation of a systemic failure to understand the true origins of most pain—in a perfect storm with unhinged corporate greed.

I find it disturbing that the medical profession is perfectly comfortable giving a sophisticated-sounding "diagnosis" to a condition without understanding its origins. Many of these diagnoses basically translate into, "You have pain in a particular region of your body, but we don't really know where it comes from." Insurance companies provide compensation and incentives to doctors for writing prescriptions. Standards of care and insurance coding accept medication as an appropriate treatment for pain, as opposed to our work, which would be categorized as massage and is marginalized. Our medical system rewards symptomatic solutions that are guaranteed to fail in a majority of cases. Misunderstanding the true origins of pain isn't simply a lost opportunity; it can have damaging, even lethal consequences.

After working on many clients with chronic pain as a Thai therapist, it became clear to me that, in most cases, dulling chronic pain with opioids was, at best, a product of misunderstanding. Whether via ignorance, ill intent, or both, millions of human beings are poorly served by the medical system. And early on as a bodyworker, I got a crash course in how many lives could be ruined as a result. Given the belief that pain is due to injury and disease, pharmaceutical and surgical interventions seem to make sense, but my explorations of bodywork, neuroscience, and trigger point therapy have told me something different.

The Culture of Powerlessness and Dependency

Any manual therapist has a ringside view of the pain epidemic. People in pain usually try more conventional methods, like seeing their family doctor, until they realize that it's a dead end and all they come away with is a prescription for painkillers for their "tendonitis" or some other disease or injury. Some might seek out more alternative approaches, such as chiropractic, acupuncture, and massage. While results are hugely variable, these people seem to find at least some relief. However, at our clinic, we routinely see patients who have been to dozens of alternative practitioners with little success. Their experiences mirror my own with recurrent, crippling back pain as a young man. I came to realize that seeing the doctor for these issues was a waste of time, and the inevitable result was a prescription for valium or NSAIDs. So, I tried many of the alternative modalities with no lasting success.

Many alternative practitioners consciously or unconsciously cultivate a dependency relationship with their patients. In so many words, they say, "I can help you as long as you come to me every week, and we can 'manage' your pain." Some therapists, and even entire professions, are fond of the dependency relationship because it seems like a good economic model, creating reliable clients who return every week. The dependency itself is insidious and disempowering—and tends to keep people in pain. In terms of the recent understanding of the biopsychosocial components of chronic pain, a mental state of empowerment and autonomy leads to far more success than feeling like a powerless victim reliant on weekly practitioner visits to avoid the risk of feeling worse.

This approach parallels what happens in the medical system. Nobody can explain why you magically develop inflammation, tendonitis, scar tissue, or the other so-called diagnoses for your pain. You get your medical description and diagnosis and take your medications—perhaps consider surgery because your body is broken. And of course, in a small minority of cases, the body is in need of invasive procedures and repair.

Personally, I was never happy with this approach, either as a patient or a practitioner. I never could quite accept that the human body was this delicate, failure-prone machine and that I needed to visit a specialist every week to keep it working. There was no real attempt to understand why I had the pain in the first place.

In my own work, I've found that the best way to empower clients to independence is to assist them in understanding the true origins of their pain. I teach my clients about what I'm doing and why. I always approach therapy as an educational exercise because huge benefits accrue when the patient begins to feel a sense of understanding, hope, and mastery. I've found this to be very successful and quite empowering to people who have been failed by many "experts."

To support this feeling, I carefully choose at-home exercises for them that further assist in lowering their pain levels. Simply moving out of the dependent victim role has a major impact in encouraging the CNS to relax its hypervigilant, protective stance.

Trigger Point Therapy: A Potential Solution

I had been practicing Thai massage for a couple of years and was searching for more knowledge when I came across Clair Davies's *Trigger Point Workbook* in 2002. By that time, I had a clear sense that my Thai education had not prepared me adequately to treat the pain conditions that my clients were coming in with. Davies's book gave me hope, and while my own work has evolved to be very different, that was my first education in how effective trigger point therapy could be.

The first key insight was simply the phenomenon of pain referral. I intuitively understood the concept that pressure on a point could cause pain somewhere else; I had seen that plenty in my own body and during my sessions. It just made sense.

An even more revolutionary core tenet of trigger point theory is that a large percentage of the pain people experience comes from muscles. This key idea was illustrated throughout Davies's book by his engaging client stories.

The enormous implication of muscles causing most pain was that most of the medical explanations people receive, even from experts, are wrong. Again, I had witnessed this with my clients. Even without trigger point knowledge, I had been able to help quite a few people, which told me that their pain wasn't originating in their torn rotator cuff, nerve impingement at the spine, carpal tunnel syndrome, and so on. I was already seriously skeptical about these diagnoses but didn't have a direction to pursue other than my own experiments.

The pain referral map from trigger point therapy provided an immediate, practical starting point in discovering an alternative explanation for pain. If a client's wrist hurt, I could explore muscles in their forearm and shoulder rather than assuming it was arthritis or tendonitis and giving up.

These ideas really excited me. They seemed to be the key I was looking for, but a few things were still missing. Davies's approach involved simple cross-fiber strokes over the trigger point area, but he didn't value stretching or movement of any kind. My training in Thai massage, on the other hand, revolved almost completely around moving the body. So, my first challenge was figuring out how to best apply my Thai techniques to trigger point therapy.

Soon after, I quickly immersed myself in the medical textbooks by Janet Travell and David Simons, the MDs who began formulating trigger point therapy in the 1940s. These monumental books provided me with a rich well of learning and still do to this day. What I didn't yet understand at the time was that this theory, in spite of its enormous value, also lacks components that prevent it from being fully realized as a therapeutic system. I'll go into that more fully in a later chapter.

At the time, these hidden stumbling blocks meant that I could help some of my people with some of their issues, but not others.

And much more often than I was happy with, their pain would return and require more therapy. As I worked with more people and my attempts to apply my newfound knowledge were hit or miss, I did begin to have some success, which made me both excited and grateful.

My encounter with Davies's brilliant book and Travell and Simons's trigger point therapy lit a spark that I knew could shine a bright light on my efforts to help people. I hoped in my modest way that I could make a difference in the crisis that was clearly developing in our medical approach to pain, and from my current perspective, I would say that hope has been gratifyingly borne out. However, if I knew then how much work it would take to get here, I might not have continued.

Naivete can be a blessing.

Client Story: Failed Back Syndrome

I was visiting Los Angeles quite a few years ago and was contacted by a woman who had found me on the web and thought I might be able to help her. As soon as I arrived and saw her shuffling to the door of her beautiful Beverly Hills home, I knew that this was a serious situation. She was accompanied by a spinal cord stimulator that she rolled alongside her body. It was supposed to send a signal to her spine that would interfere with her incessant and constant pain.

She handed me a stack of medical records a foot high as I was to begin our two-hour session. It was early in my career, and I was far less confident than I am today in my ability to help her in the face of this wall of medical records. I felt compassion for this woman, barely in her fifties, who, in spite of being able to afford the best medical care, was clearly en route to complete disability. The implant was losing its effectiveness, and her doctors were proposing the next escalation: a pain pump, which would provide a steady stream of opioid medication to her body. She said that she feared being in a wheelchair in the not too distant future.

Her story was a textbook example of the cascading damage that can happen when surgeries go bad. Her condition began with a bike accident when she was a girl. She broke her collarbone and underwent the first of what became seven or eight surgeries by the time I met her. Each surgery brought with it another setback, and the last several were back surgeries. She had many diagnoses, among them "failed back surgery syndrome." This term is unique in the medical profession, as there is no equivalent term for other types of failed surgeries. It simply refers to the unfortunately very common occurrence that a patient's pain is not alleviated by their back surgery.[8]

Fortunately, by the time I met with her, I had enough success with my approach that I decided to put the stack of medical records down, along with my fear, and do a treatment with her. Her primary complaint was constant, severe pain radiating down her leg from her hip and low back. Even with the implant device, she was finding sleep difficult. This pain pattern is very common and something that we routinely treat with success. Two muscles in the lower back and hips generally set up that type of pain: quadratus lumborum (QL) and gluteus minimus.

At the beginning of the session, she could hardly let me touch her. Anyone who has been in that much pain for that long develops a highly upregulated (sensitized) and protective emotional posture, considering any input to be threatening. And this is half the problem, as I will expand upon later. So our first test and opportunity is to earn trust and create some experiences of movement with less pain.

I made my movements very slow and small. When she would seize and flinch, I would have her take a breath and continue to move her, providing manual feedback over the areas that were presenting as the most painful. This approach distracts the CNS from the experience of pain, causing it to relax a small bit of its control and protective engagement of the muscles.

---

8   Peter Ullrich, "Failed Back Surgery Syndrome (FBSS): What It Is and How to Avoid Pain after Surgery," *Spine-health*, November 4, 2009, https://www.spine-health.com/treatment/back-surgery/failed-back-surgery-syndrome-fbss-what-it-and-how-avoid-pain-after-surgery.

I knew that her symptoms, while presenting in a frighteningly severe and overwhelming package, were most likely from the same soft-tissue source as the hundreds of milder cases we had treated successfully. Ultimately, most non-acute pain arises from the CNS and how it responds to muscular signals.

Over time and the cascading effects of surgeries to fix failed surgeries, her CNS had decided that complete protective engagement was necessary to keep her safe and intact. My job was to convince it that at least some of the danger it was perceiving was not actually present, with evidence in the form of very small, incremental improvements as we moved her and she experienced less and less pain. We call this "pain hacking."

Before long, she was beginning to move more freely, and I could apply more direct pressure to her QL and gluteal muscles as I helped her increase the range of motion in her leg. Beginning with passive movements, I had her become increasingly active as her CNS benefitted from the positive effects of witnessing the return of movement without pain.

My own fear and anxiety began to lessen as I realized that this poor woman who had been dealt a terribly unfortunate medical hand was responding to my work in the same way as hundreds of others with far less severe issues. The foot-high stack of medical records notwithstanding, she began to let go and move without pain. In spite of the daunting circumstances, the model held, and I could feel her tangible relief as the session went on.

She wrote me the next day and told me that not only was I the first manual therapist who hadn't made her pain worse, but she was experiencing an overall reduction in pain of 80 percent, and not just in her leg. It seemed like magic, except that I had seen this arc many times before, just not as vividly.

This experience obviously made me very happy—and also a little sad. Had we met much earlier in her history, what might have happened? And what about the millions of individuals who are being victimized by our ongoing state of ignorance about the true origins and appropriate treatments for pain?

Back Surgery for Back Pain: A Surgeon's View

Failed back surgery syndrome is so common that it has its own insurance code. The statistics in back surgery are truly horrifying.[9] Each successive surgery doubles the likelihood of failure. Nowhere does the misunderstanding of the role of injury and disease in pain have greater impact than in the world of spinal surgery. My friend Dr. David Hanscom, author of the books *Back In Control* and *Do You Really Need Spine Surgery,*[10] is a prominent spinal surgeon who began to realize that his profession was grossly irresponsible in its treatment of back pain. He made the statement in a conversation we had a couple of years ago that "back surgery doesn't fix back pain."

He showed me several X-rays of individuals in which extensive spinal fusions had been done by other surgeons to supposedly address moderate amounts of back pain. One women's entire spine was fused after complaining about relatively moderate, short-term thoracic pain. The results were so damaging to her physically and psychologically that she became psychotic. Dr. Hanscom eventually left the profession and now devotes his impressive work to research in downregulation of the nervous system as a way to treat intractable chronic pain.

---

9   David Hanscom, *Back in Control: A Surgeon's Roadmap Out of Chronic Pain, 2nd Edition* (Vertus Press, 2016).

10 David Hanscom, *Do You Really Need Spine Surgery? Take Control with a Surgeon's Advice* (Vertus Press, 2019).

"A client came to me for work on the table. She was having breathing issues, and her doctor had recommended massage on her trapezius to relieve 'pressure on her lungs.' I explained my CTB approach and what I believed the issue could be, but to soothe her mind, I also appeased the doctor's orders and worked on her back first.

"She had had Covid the month prior, during which she coughed quite a bit. She was having a hard time breathing, her chest felt tight, and she was experiencing pain near her breast that made her feel like she had heart problems, which is a classic pectoralis major symptom.

"I focused on her clavicular pec major and pec minor using the CTB Upper Core Protocol. The pain went away immediately after working these areas. I explained how to continue treating those areas at home, and she booked a mat session to address what she thought was a pulled hamstring. Knowing that hamstring issues are usually due to posterior gluteus minimus referral, I worked on her with parts of the Lower Core Protocol, and she was able to do her yoga practice and stretch normally, without pain. The next day, she told me I was 'her new doctor' and that her pain had resolved. She was very happy to find that it was all muscular and not her heart or lungs."

—Jodi Fritts, LMT, CTB practitioner

CHAPTER 3

The New Science of Pain

Recent neuroscience has shown us that many of the embedded beliefs about the nature and origins of pain in our medical system are simply wrong. In this chapter, I'll provide a brief summary of the history of pain theories and highlight some exciting new developments in neuroscience that underpin my work.

At the heart of the medical system's abject failure to adequately diagnose and treat pain is an old, embedded belief that pain is something that just happens to us, a force from the outside. This notion dates back hundreds of years. Prior to the Renaissance, it was believed that pain existed outside of the body, possibly as a redemptive punishment from God, as in the example of Jesus on the cross.

In his monumental *Treatise on Man* (1664), René Descartes updated this idea somewhat by proposing that the body was like a machine with vessels that could conduct pain from outside the body to the brain. Descartes introduced the concept that the brain perceived pain, but that pain still existed independently as a physical existence. Pain could be mediated by cutting the fibers that transmitted pain into the organism.

While neuroscience has progressed considerably since Descartes and has invalidated his idea, the belief in pain as an external force persists in modern medical culture. This is basically the underlying belief behind "injury-centric thinking." The injury or inflammation causes the pain, so the misguided conclusion is to always look for the injury at the site where the patient perceives their pain.

Some Historical Pain Theories

In the 1800s, German physiologist Johannes P. Müller developed the concept of sensory nerve specificity or the "law of specific nerve energies." His ideas became known as *specificity theory*, which proposed that there were specific receptors devoted to the "sensation" of pain. This basically put an end to the idea that there was a physical property of the sensation being carried into the brain, as Descartes had postulated. However, while receptors for pressure, vibration, heat, and cold were discovered, pain receptors were never isolated in the body. The idea of specific pain receptors persisted for a long time, mostly among physiologists, but eventually gave way to an understanding that pain is different than sensation and fabricated somewhere along the pathway of the nervous system. Specificity theory was slowly displaced by intensity theory.[11]

In 1874, German neurologist Wilhelm Heinrich Erb proposed the *intensity theory* of pain, which claimed that the sensation of pain was related to the intensity of the stimulus. Weak stimuli produce nonpainful sensations, while stronger stimuli produce pain.

Over a decade later, in 1889, German physiologist Bernhard Naunyn conducted a compelling series of experiments in which he rapidly prodded the skin of a patient with an imperceivable stimulus such as the touch of a human hair (60–600 times per second). After 6–20 seconds, the patient reported unbearable pain. This is a fascinating study for many reasons. The stimulus was very localized, below the level of

11 Jun Chen, "History of Pain Theories," *Neuroscience Bulletin* 27, no. 5 (September 29, 2011): 344–6, https://doi.org/10.1007/s12264-011-0139-0.

perception, but it was repetitive and exposed the sensors to a microscopic stimulus many times in rapid succession. There was certainly no level of tissue injury, excessive heat or cold, or pressure involved. Yet the response of the system was a perception of unbearable pain.[12]

Naunyn's experiments completely decoupled the experience of severe pain from tissue damage. They showed that the CNS is capable of generating an experience of unbearable pain on the basis of an imperceptible input—in this case, the touch of a human hair. Yet our current medical system retains the physical model of pain proposed by Descartes in its relentless focus on disease and injury behind any report of pain. There is always an attempt to find the physical origin of the pain, only instead of a hot fire, it presumes tissue damage as the source.

Gate control theory, proposed by Ronald Melzack and Patrick Wall in 1965, attempts to provide a completely physiological explanation for pain phenomena by postulating two types of nerve fibers whose interaction controls the intensity of pain: a thin (pain) fiber and a large diameter fiber. Their model tries to provide a physical explanation for what was emerging as a psychological component of the pain response. This model has proven to be overly simplistic and, in some aspects, physiologically incorrect in its attempt to physicalize what has emerged as a far richer "biopsychosocial" understanding of pain.

Current pain theory recognizes that pain is an output, not an input. Pain is a sensation produced by the brain, based upon many inputs, including but not limited to nociception, or danger signals, from monitoring sensors embedded throughout the body.

Pain versus Nociception

The term *nociception* was coined by the British neurophysiologist Sir Charles Scott Sherrington in 1900 to distinguish the

---

12 Chen, "History of Pain Theories," 346.

experience of pain, which was, by then, recognized as a subjective phenomenon from the physiological signaling of danger and local disturbance. Nociceptors provide input the CNS uses to protect the body from injury. This is an extremely important concept. A nociceptor is like the oil light in your car. It provides you, the driver, with important information about your ability to operate the car safely. However, it doesn't determine your actions. You might decide to immediately stop and add oil, or you might choose to ignore it. And sometimes, the light itself is faulty, and your car still has plenty of oil.

We have *nociceptive organs* that are sensitive to mechanical pressure, excessive heat, and certain chemicals. Dangerous levels of these phenomena are transmitted as nociceptive signals to the CNS. It's then up to the brain to decide what to do about it, including the potential generation of pain. In the case of an acute injury involving tissue damage, it is quite likely that an experience of pain will result due to the nociceptive compounds generated at the site of the injury. This leads us to a strong association between injury and pain, but they are not the same.

Dr. Lorimer Mosely, professor of clinical neurosciences and chair in physiotherapy at the Sansom Institute for Health Research at the University of South Australia, says, "Pain is the output. Nociception is one of the inputs. All of the inputs are evaluated when we're talking about pain, I think, according to this question: how dangerous is this? Based on everything I know, which is all of the information available to me right now, how dangerous is this really?"[13] According to Mosely, nociception is not the only input processed by the CNS, although it is certainly a very important one. The CNS also processes

---

13 Nils Oudhuis, "50 Shades of Pain With Prof. Lorimer Moseley," Trust Me, I'm a Physiotherapist, May 20, 2017, https://trustmephysiotherapy.com/50-shades-of-pain-with-lorimer-moseley.

emotions, stress, and the environment, and the brain integrates and interprets these stimuli.

Basically, pain is a survival mechanism. It is like that smoke alarm in your house, making a loud, annoying noise to tell you something is wrong, whether there's a real house fire or just a pizza cooking in the oven.

But there's another curious aspect to how we perceive pain. Dr. Mosely found that soft tissue damage and nociception are *neither necessary nor sufficient* for the experience of pain. Someone can have major tissue damage and feel nothing at all. A soldier can have a limb blown off and feel nothing until out of harm's way.

With that in mind, we must understand that most chronic pain has little or nothing to do with tissue damage, a topic that we will explore in more detail shortly.

Before we continue, we must take a look at how the brain reacts to pain.

Neuroplasticity: How the Brain Adapts to Change

At one time, neuroscientists thought that once childhood development had finished, the brain could no longer do anything but decline and lose neurons. Once a neuron died, so it was thought, that neuron could never be regenerated. While we readily accept that the brain changes in response to cognitive learning, it was much slower to change the belief that areas of the brain that control physical processes are hardwired. In fact, the CNS has an astonishing ability to rewire itself on the fly, within minutes, a characteristic called *neuroplasticity*.

In the 1960s, neuroscientist Michael Merzenich made some of the earliest discoveries of adult plasticity. Prior to that time, most scientists believed that there was a fixed region of the brain devoted to each specific activity, such as moving a specific finger, being touched on a leg, seeing with each eye, and so on, which they called *localizationism*.

Quite accidentally, Merzenich found hard evidence that the brain is fluid and can remap and reuse its precious neuronal territory. For example, if a finger had been amputated, the area of the brain that controlled that finger would not go to waste; it would be remapped to handle the processing of the remaining fingers. Contrary to the prevailing belief, he discovered that the adult brain constantly refines its maps and connections to sensory and motor control of the body based on the learning that occurs via repetitive tasks.

Merzenich, in his later work, has used these discoveries to facilitate brain remapping in children with disabilities in learning, speech recognition, attention, and focus. He found that the reorganization triggered by his language recognition training also had much broader benefits, such as increased IQ.[14]

If we imagine the body to be a computer, scientists now had to think of the brain's internal neuronal organization as *software* rather than *hardware*. If the lunar lander malfunctions, engineers on Earth can upload a new version of its programming and fix it. If those instructions were wired into silicon, it wouldn't be changeable, and the experiment would be over. Thankfully, the brain is reprogrammable, and the experiment doesn't have to end in disaster—or chronic pain.

Chronic Pain: The Dark Side of Neuroplastic Change

The exact qualities of neuroplastic change that benefit us in so many ways have a serious negative side when it comes to pain, as seen with

---

14 For an entertaining and accessible look at neuroplasticity, I recommend Norman Doidge, *The Brain That Changes Itself: Stories of Personal Triumph from the Frontiers of Brain Science* (New York: Penguin Books, 2007).

phantom limb pain. Ninety-five percent of amputees experience an ongoing sensation of the limb still being present and actually feel pain in the area where the limb would have been. In some cases, this can become a horribly disturbing way to live, even leading to suicide.

Neuroscientist V. S. Ramachandran, in a brilliant leap, posited that the brain's map for the missing limb was disturbed because the limb could no longer be moved or provide proprioceptive input to the brain. Basically, the brain remained "stuck" in the injured state of the arm pre-amputation. So, he hypothesized that if he could trick the brain into believing that the limb was still attached, he could help a patient find relief.

Ramachandran devised an experiment in which he used a simple mirror that gave the brain the illusion that the missing limb was present and healthy. His hope was that by processing this visual information, it would lead the brain to neuroplastic change, correcting its own model of the arm as a working, intact limb and alleviating the experience of pain. This classic example of a neurological hack (again, the computer analogy) was extremely successful, and he was permanently able to eliminate the phantom pain in some of his patients, as long as they stuck with it for a period of weeks or months.

Building on this work, Ramachandran set out to study a condition called reflex sympathetic dystrophy, in which following a nociceptive event such as a sting or bruise, the body falls into a state of "guarding." It retains a strong memory of the pain so that even the lightest touch can trigger it again. In order to protect against further injury, the brain actually triggers the pain moments before the limb is moved, which then essentially immobilizes it. As a protective response to actual injury, this makes sense. If you broke your arm, you would want to splint and immobilize it to prevent further tissue damage from occurring. However, sometimes when a perceived injury is no longer there, the brain gets stuck in the model it constructed at the time of the original nociceptive event.

He used the mirror box with his amputee patients and was able to give some of them relief just by seeing the reflection of their good arm moving normally without pain. Ramachandran harnessed the power of neuroplasticity to substitute a new map of the arm that didn't include its injury, now healed, and the patients' pain disappeared. Ramachandran was the first major researcher to posit that the brain controls the sensation of pain, "an opinion on the organism's response to health rather than a reflexive response to injury."[15]

In his model, the brain constructs a virtual reality model of the body and determines whether pain is an appropriate response. However, like a software program, the brain's output is only as good as its inputs. When the inputs are disturbed with a dramatic event such as an amputation (or when, as I will argue later, the brain is presented with steady nociception from trigger points), its map of the body is going to become faulty.

Dr. Moseley thought he might be able to add another dimension to the experiment by further enhancing the construction of a new mental map. In addition to the mirror therapy, he showed patients images of hands and had them participate in visualization exercises. Many of these long-term patients recovered with Moseley's protocol.[16]

These two scientists proved that if you have an actual injury, it will generate a strong stream of nociception to the brain, and you

---

15 Norman Doidge, *The Brain That Changes Itself: Stories of Personal Triumph from the Frontiers of Brain Science*, (New York: Penguin Books, 2014), 151.

16 Moseley tells a story in his excellent and entertaining TED Talk on pain. He was walking in the bush, felt something brush his leg, and thought nothing of it until his leg started to swell and become painful. He realized he had been bitten by a venomous adder and needed a hospital. The bite was quite serious and painful. Many years later, he was walking and something brushed against his leg. A jolt of searing pain shot up his leg, but it was only a branch. A similar stimulus in the same area of his leg triggered the brain's internally stored model of that event and it triggered the same pain in response. Lorimer Mosely, "Why Things Hurt," filmed November 2011 at TEDxAdelaide, video, 14:32, https://www.youtube.com/watch?v=gwd-wLdIHjs.

are likely to experience pain. Even in circumstances like this, the brain may decide not to generate pain due to its assessment of the overall state of the organism. An injury involving tissue damage can heal completely in a few weeks, at which point, theoretically, the pain should stop. Unfortunately, a significant number of people develop chronic pain despite the original injury being healed. In these cases, the brain's internal model got stuck and memorized the state of affairs at the time of the injury.

Central Downregulation: Remapping the Virtual Body

If the brain can change itself, then we can find ways to reprogram it from chronic pain to relief. This process is called downregulation. But how do we get there?

Michael Moskowitz, MD, has devoted his career to understanding how neuroplasticity works with chronic pain. His work focuses on *central downregulation*: using various techniques to assist his patients in changing their brain's inner model.[17] He began his investigations in an effort to alleviate his own chronic pain from two major injuries. To treat his own pain, Moskowitz invented visualization exercises for himself in which he saw the expanded brain maps shrinking and normalizing. Over a period of months, he eliminated his own chronic pain.

In his experience, he observed a principle of modern neuroscience: "what fires together wires together." Once pain is initiated with a significant nociceptive event, the brain turns on more receptors—upregulates—and makes the nervous system more sensitive to nociceptive input. This process occurs in any kind of learning, but

---

17 Moskowitz runs a clinic in Sausalito, California, where he treats truly desperate chronic pain patients who have been abandoned by conventional medicine. He is having significant success in an area that is considered untreatable with conventional techniques.

when pain is involved, the results are insidious. At the very time when we hope to begin the process of repair, desensitization, and pain relief, the body turns up its sensitivity via neuroplastic change. At the same time that sensitivity increases, the brain expands its virtual map to assign more neurons to sensations from that part of the body.

This is what ultimately happens with phantom limb pain. The intense nociception from the injured limb causes this upregulation and distortion of the inner mapping, which persists even when the limb is gone. The limb doesn't cause the pain; the traumatic load of danger signals from the injury or disease has caused neuroplastic changes that become dissociated from the actual condition of the body. The brain, in a somewhat flawed attempt at self-preservation, decides to produce pain as an output based on this errant internal map. This process makes chronic pain extremely difficult to treat with medication because it's no longer a matter of interrupting peripheral nociceptive signals unless the person has trigger points that are generating nociception related to that area. This is quite possible because trigger points are not on the radar of most central downregulation practitioners.

Other strategies for central downregulation—such as writing, meditation, and so on—are effective, but they require discipline and motivation from the patient over a period of months in most cases to get solid results. Addressing relevant trigger points could greatly speed up this process. In the next section, I explain why trigger points work, taking satellite referral into account, should be included as an important aspect of treatment.

Trigger Points: The Missing Link for Neuroplastic Change

To date, neuroscientists using neuroplasticity to treat chronic pain have mostly focused on the downregulation and remapping of the CNS, remodeling the mind's virtual map of the body, releasing unconscious emotional content, and downregulating its sensitivity to inputs. There has been no real focus on the peripheral, and for good reason. If we assume that there was originally an injury, surgery, or other traumatic event that produced a cascade of nociceptive input, after a period of time, the injury will have healed, and the nociceptive stream from the periphery is no longer coming in. In the case of phantom limb pain, the limb is literally gone. The problem is that the brain remembers the state of the limb from before—when there was an actual, vivid, severe injury or disease. In this model, it would make little sense to focus on the periphery because the central changes and remapping in the brain are now considered to be responsible for the pain.

In my own work, I've focused on what I believe is a huge missing element in this model: the role of trigger points as peripheral sources of ongoing nociception. There is, for the most part, a gaping divide between the community of trigger point researchers and more mainstream science. While the neuroscientists I've highlighted above are doing groundbreaking work, there has been little to no attention paid to trigger points as peripheral sources of nociception and sensitization. However, several trigger point researchers have made their own groundbreaking and revelatory discoveries.

The authors and editors of the third edition of *Travell, Simons & Simons' Myofascial Pain and Dysfunction: The Trigger Point Manual* have concluded that in the absence of tissue damage, trigger points "function as persistent sources of nociceptive input and contribute to peripheral and central sensitization," as well as neuroplastic change characteristic of chronic pain.[18]

Dr. Jay Shah of the National Institutes of Health has devoted his career to understanding the physiology of trigger points and how

18 Joseph M. Donnelly, et al., *Travell, Simons & Simons' Myofascial Pain and Dysfunction: The Trigger Point Manual, Third Edition*, (Philadelphia: Wolters Kluwer, 2019), 102.

they interact with the CNS. Using microtubules—essentially hollow acupuncture needles—he has sampled the chemical milieu of trigger points in muscle and discovered excess concentrations of several inflammatory compounds known to stimulate muscle nociceptors in both active and latent trigger points.[19] These chemicals—such as cytokines, 5-HT, CGRP, IL-6, IL-8, and others—typically indicate an inflammatory response to injury. When muscular nociceptors detect inflammatory chemicals, they pass that information to the CNS, which interprets the signal as injury and outputs a pain response.

Yet, in the case of trigger points and amputee patients, injury is no longer present. Trigger points aren't injuries; they are cell-level disturbances that are often easily cleared by the body, but not always. However, the presence of inflammatory chemicals creates a sort of "false flag" operation in the body and causes the brain to operate as if there is some level of ongoing injury or disease.

Trigger points are an active source of nociception that aren't an injury, and they set up central sensitization and changes in the brain's mapping—everything that is needed to set up chronic pain. When a trigger point persists over a long period of time (which, without intervention, can easily be years or decades), it is a hidden transmitter, beaming nociceptive danger signals to the CNS and giving the danger assessment apparatus something to very correctly be concerned with. The brain is simply doing its job of "Protector in Chief," and chronic pain is a rational response to this steady but hidden stream of nociception.

That said, very few people even consider the possibility that trigger points could be an ongoing nociceptive source. This is

19 Jay P. Shah and Elizabeth A. Gilliams, "Uncovering the Biochemical Milieu of Myofascial Trigger Points Using in Vivo Microdialysis: An Application of Muscle Pain Concepts to Myofascial Pain Syndrome," *Journal of Bodywork and Movement Therapies,* 12, no. 4 (2008), doi:10.1016/j.jbmt.2008.06.006.

likely because of a persistent and deep bias among many in the medical community that trigger point therapy—as first described by Travell and Simons—is "soft science" and passé, even though research by Shah and other devoted researchers fits perfectly with the most recent discoveries in neuroscience.

But how do trigger points develop in the first place, especially if they can cause so much pain and dysfunction in the body? In the next chapter, we will cover the origins and behavior of trigger points.

"I've seen many people who experience headaches and generalized shoulder pain and many who have been diagnosed with rotator cuff tears and similar injuries. One client story, in particular, demonstrates the power of the protocols and techniques taught in the Coaching the Body training and how they not only restore mobility and decrease pain but also empower people to take their wellness into their own hands and better understand their bodies and relationship to pain.

"Jeff is a hardworking carpenter with a physically demanding lifestyle. He was referred to me by a mutual friend who he had been talking with about his ongoing shoulder pain and its detrimental effect on his ability to work. Jeff wasn't the type to receive bodywork, though he had regularly seen a chiropractor for many years. We scheduled a phone conversation, and it's safe to say he was a skeptic at best. With a little encouragement, he came in to give the CTB modality a try. He reported pain in nearly all parts of his shoulder, he had three confirmed rotator cuff tears, and his range of motion was limited to around 60 degrees. These limits left him struggling to work and live the active lifestyle he enjoyed.

"Knowing his uncertainty, we scheduled a forty-five-minute intro session 'just to see how it goes.' Upon arrival, he showed me his range and how far he could lift his arm without pain. He was very limited, and it was easy to see why he was willing to try just about anything so that he could continue to work until his inevitable surgery. I kept the session very basic, focusing on the CTB Scapular Positioning Protocol, and engaged with him throughout, tracking his felt experience. Jeff intuitively understood body awareness and cooperation and was able to make the most of the contract/relax exercises. He met me in the waiting room after the session, and when I asked him to try out his range, he lifted his arm well past 90 degrees and reported no pain. It was like magic!

"I continued to see him up to his surgery date, keeping him mobile and working. We started back up very soon after this surgery, working in tandem with his physical therapy. The tears were very real, but as I had learned in my training, freeing up scapular movement can very often lessen pain and restore range without the surgical interventions. Jeff continues to work, farm, and ranch, and I still see him on a regular basis both for lower body and upper body care. More recently, he's been dealing with back pain that affects his hips, legs, and knee and was diagnosed with severe stenosis. Through continued sessions and regular independent self-care, he's slowly tapered off the gabapentin and continues to live his life at top speed, just the way he likes it."

—Kelly Harris, CTB practitioner and yoga instructor,

Quad Cities, Iowa

CHAPTER 4

What Are Trigger Points?

Before we go any further, we must first understand the origins of trigger point therapy and its limitations, as well as the nature of trigger points and how they cause pain and discomfort in the body.

Early Understanding of Trigger Points

Trigger points have been observed and written about for centuries, starting in the sixteenth century, but the idea that they cause a significant percentage of commonly experienced pain has achieved little acceptance in the medical community. Over one hundred years ago, researchers observed what they called "thickenings" or "muscle callouses" in an attempt to describe what we now know as *taut fibers*.[20] In spite of great advances in understanding these fibers as actually originating from a type of contraction, most therapists are still taught to think of the ropey fibers in muscle as "scar tissue" or "adhesions." Yet, trigger point therapists know that these hard fibers can often be softened and even eliminated in a matter of minutes, which would be physiologically impossible if

---

20 Jay P. Shah, et al., "Myofascial Trigger Points Then and Now: A Historical and Scientific Perspective," *PM&R: The Journal of Injury, Function and Rehabilitation* 7, no. 7 (2015): 746–761, https://pubmed.ncbi.nlm.nih.gov/25724849/.

they were composed of thickened connective tissue. Unless there was some form of gross trauma, these hard fibers are not likely from scar tissue. In fact, hard fibers are the first thing we look for when examining a muscle for trigger points.

In the 1940s, physician Janet Travell came across the work of J. H. Kellgren, who was experimenting with inducing pain referral via saline injection, while working in a cardiac clinic at Sea View Hospital in Staten Island. She observed that many of her pulmonary disease patients had devastating pain in their shoulders and arms. She found that there were hard areas of muscle in their chest and scapular areas that, when manually compressed, reproduced the patients' pain. Soon after, she learned that doctors Arthur Steindler and J. V. Luck from the University of Iowa had been experimenting with injecting procaine hydrochloride into the hard muscle areas, which offered patients some degree of pain relief.[21]

Later, Travell herself began to have shoulder pain that bothered her while playing tennis. In an effort to relieve the pain, her father injected procaine into a tender spot in the infraspinatus muscle (in the back of her shoulder). The pain went away, and being very intrigued, Travell wrote her first paper on trigger points in 1942.[22] Ten years later, she wrote a paper covering the referred pain patterns of thirty-two muscles, which quickly became a classic reference on the subject of myofascial pain.[23]

---

21 Larry W. White and Janet G. Travell, "Janet G. Travell, MD on Myofascial Pain," *Journal of Clinical Orthodontics*, (July 1989) https://www.jco-online.com/archive/1989/07/468-jco-interviews-janet-g-travell-md-on-myofascial-pain.

22 Janet Travell, et al., "Pain and Disability of the Shoulder and Arm: Treatment by Intramuscular Infiltration with Procaine Hydrochloride," *Journal of the American Medical Association* 120, no. 6 (1942): 417–422, doi:10.1001/jama.1942 .02830410005002.

23 Janet Travell and Seymour H. Rinzler, "The Myofascial Genesis of Pain," *Postgraduate Medicine* 11, no. 5 (May 1952): 425–34, https://doi.org/10.1080/00325481.1952 .11694280.

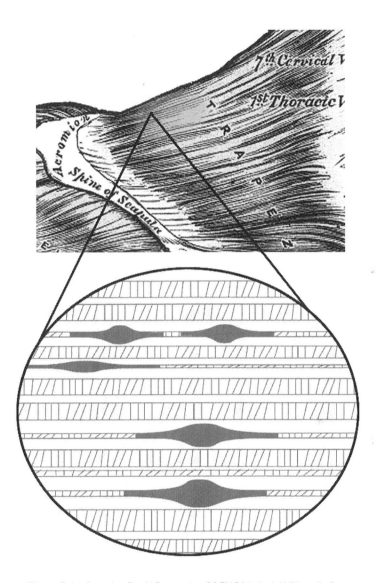

Fig. 4-1. Trigger Point Complex. David Parmenter, CC BY-SA 3.0, via Wikimedia Commons.

Travell achieved a tremendous amount in the field, including becoming John F. Kennedy's White House Physician and allowing him to carry on with his political career without debilitating pain; in 1982, she wrote a two-volume reference, *Myofascial Pain and*

Dysfunction: The Trigger Point Manual, with David Simons. But the book was written for MDs, and as such, the procedures—injection and using a cold spray (ethyl chloride) only available to medical personnel—were technical and required professional application.

Almost two decades later, in 2001, Clair Davies wrote *The Trigger Point Therapy Workbook: Your Self-Treatment Guide for Pain Relief*. Davies applied Travell and Simons's material by developing massage-based self-care approaches to common pain conditions. He was an engaging, sincere man who had a deep respect for the work of Travell and Simons and set out to apply it as a self-care technique. His lively storytelling, warmth, and humor made scientific and technical concepts fun and easy to understand.

The Trigger Point Therapy Workbook singlehandedly brought Travell and Simons's concepts to the general reader, transcending the narrow medical genre to which they had been confined. Fortunately, I encountered his book in a Borders Bookstore in 2001.

The Trigger Point Model

From a macro perspective, myofascial trigger points, or MTrPs, are areas of spot tenderness in a palpable taut band of muscle fiber. They are called "trigger points" because they trigger pain and other sensations in distant parts of the body, a phenomenon called "referral." The term "point" is misleading in this context. You cannot discern individual points, only bundles of many hardened muscle fibers that feel more like a tube or rope than a point. These are the result of microphysiological events that have happened over a region of a muscle, involving hundreds or thousands of individual fibers.

In the region of the trigger point, a group of tense muscle fibers extends from the trigger point to muscle attachments. This group of tense muscle fibers is a *taut band*. The increased tension of the taut bands is caused by regional shortening of the sarcomeres (the smallest unit of muscle tissue). So, what we call a point could be more accurately described as a trigger point complex.

The taut band will have a tender area somewhere along its length, generally near the neuromuscular junction in the motor endplate zone (where the motor nerve joins the muscle). In a particular fiber, the motor endplate zone will be located near the center of that fiber. Finding taut bands is the first step in locating a trigger point. Anywhere you feel hard, taut fibers, you are likely to find tenderness near the endplate zone.

What Is a Taut Fiber?

A taut fiber might feel like scar tissue, but it's very different. Fibers with trigger points go into *contracture*. This is different than contraction.

Contraction involves the entire muscle and is an active response to an external signal from a motor nerve. Energy input is necessary to maintain the contraction. Muscle fibers consist of two parts that can slide together, like a curtain and rod. A muscle contracts by its fibers sliding together in response to a motor signal. To accomplish this, adenosine triphosphate (ATP) and free calcium (Ca++) activate the cross bridges of the myosin (motor proteins) to tug on the actin (another protein) filaments.

A *contracture*, on the other hand, happens when the sliding filaments get stuck in the fully slid-together and shortened state because of a microscopic area of stagnation in the fiber. The trigger point area in the center of the muscle fiber pulls the sarcomeres in from either end, like tying a knot in the center of a clothesline. The fibers get stuck because the particular area of the muscle is unable to provide the ATP (energy) required to move the bonds and release the fiber. Unlike a contraction, which requires ATP to stay short, a contracture will remain shortened without any further energy input. This characteristic is key.

The late Dr. Leon Chaitow pointed out that contractures could serve a useful purpose. Putting more tension into a muscle fiber is a sustainable way to provide more stability. And stability is a good thing because a stable joint is less prone to injury. This concept has become a core part of my model after working with it for many years. I truly believe that the body has an innate intelligence and logic, and if we can get inside that as therapists, we can be effective advocates. More about this idea in Chapter 7.

Tenderness

Unlike an acute injury, tenderness at trigger point locations is felt only when the area is compressed. If the trigger point is active, the client would feel pain both at rest and when being palpated. The pain is experienced in the *referred pain region* of the trigger point, which is generally at a different location. Often, the client won't feel tenderness during initial palpation, possibly because the surrounding tissues are hardened and make it difficult to localize specific taut fibers.

Another important characteristic of trigger points is that tenderness drops off dramatically as we move even a short distance away from the trigger point zone. Local tenderness is produced by nociceptive chemicals in the immediate region of the trigger point. For these reasons, it's much easier to palpate for hard bands of tissue than it is to look for tenderness. I recommend that students first find hard fibers, and after some initial palpation and treatment, tenderness is likely to be more evident in the motor endplate zone of each fiber bundle.

The Importance of Fiber Direction and Extent

Because trigger points tend to occur in the motor endplate zone of each fiber, we must understand the fiber architecture of each part of the muscle to accurately palpate for trigger points.

Muscles have varying shapes, configurations, and fiber directions depending on what function they perform. While the overall purpose of muscles is to contract, muscles must fulfill specific functions, such as bending the elbow or dorsiflexing the foot. The various muscle shapes are an excellent example of the great Chicago School architect Louis Sullivan's concept that "form follows function." While in architecture, there have been plenty of fanciful, impractical designs, we don't tend to see this as much in biology. Living organisms must practically compete and survive, and they have developed sophisticated structural adaptations to facilitate their ability to do so.

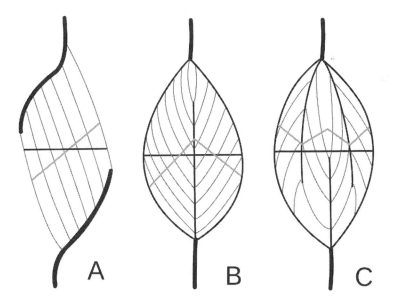

Fig 4-2. Schematic Diagram of pennate muscles, showing typical motor endplate zones at right angle to fiber direction. By Uwe Gille, own work, CC BY-SA 3.0, https://commons.wikimedia.org/w/index.php?curid=3181778.

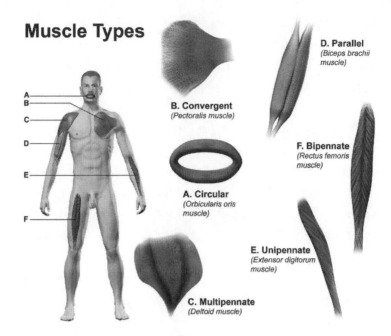

Muscle Types

D. Parallel
(Biceps brachii muscle)

B. Convergent
(Pectoralis muscle)

F. Bipennate
(Rectus femoris muscle)

A. Circular
(Orbicularis oris muscle)

E. Unipennate
(Extensor digitorum muscle)

C. Multipennate
(Deltoid muscle)

Fig. 4-3. Fusiform, pennate, and multipennate muscle shapes with motor endplate zones schematically indicated. Henry Vandyke Carter, public domain, via Wikimedia Commons.

Muscles with longitudinal fibers (also called fusiform or parallel), such as in the biceps, produce high-speed length change but tend to be weaker than muscles with oblique fibers (called pennate, meaning feather-like), such as in the rectus femoris, which are more powerful and use a lot of fibers to produce relatively small change in length. Multipennate shapes (a symmetrical feather-like shape) are seen in power muscles, such as the lateral deltoid, and are optimized to provide force during abduction of the arm.

These muscles might look similar from a distance in their overall shape, but fiber direction dramatically changes how we understand the muscle's function, the location of its endplate zones, and how we would palpate it. We always palpate fibers at right angles to their direction; this is the only way to discern differences between fiber bundles. Endplate zones tend to be near the center point between a particular fiber's transition into tendinous connective tissue. You cannot simply look at a muscle and determine where the fiber centerline is without knowing its fiber direction.

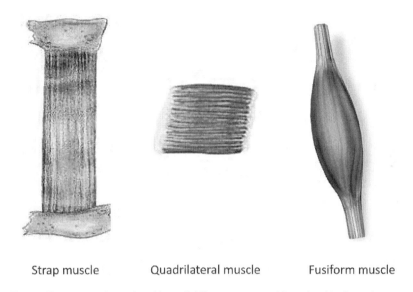

Strap muscle   Quadrilateral muscle   Fusiform muscle

Fig. 4-4. Three types of muscles with parallel fibers—strap, quadrilateral and fusiform shapes.

Pain Referral

Trigger points make the muscle sensitive to increased muscle tension, which painfully limits stretch and range of motion, and it inhibits contraction and passive shortening of the muscle. Trigger points cause region-specific pain rather than widespread, general pain. But pain is rarely felt in the area of the trigger point complex itself (less than 20 percent of the time) and is more often felt somewhere else in the body.

We often refer to this phenomenon as "referred pain," but "referred sensation" would be more accurate. It may be felt as many different qualities of pain—numbness, tingling, hot or cold—or a feeling of shakiness, weakness, or instability. At times the pain sensation may be as intense as any injury, or it could be more achy, dull, and generalized. Either way, these referred sensations follow predictable patterns specific to each muscle. These patterns also tend to be similar between individuals, with inevitable and sometimes significant variations. Because the actual experience of pain is generated by the CNS, normal variations between individuals are common.

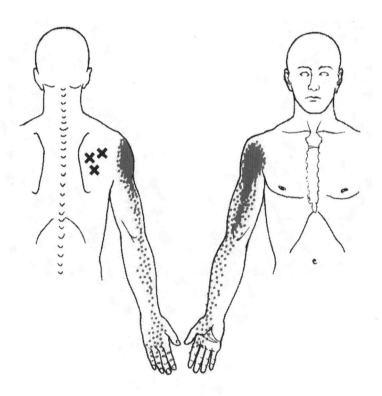

Fig. 4-5. Pain referral pattern of the infraspinatus muscle. Trigger point areas are marked with Xs.

After decades of clinical observation, Travell and Simons developed extensive pain referral drawings documenting the pain that a typical patient perceives in response to trigger point stimulation.[24] By studying several individuals for each muscle, they were able to plot where the pain was likely to occur. In the case of the infraspinatus (see Figure 4.5), the pain occurs in the front of the shoulder and down the arm. It's important to understand that the Xs in pain referral charts are only examples because trigger point areas can occur along the entire area of the endplate zones.

Muscles may only refer pain intermittently. Pain may only appear once the nociception (danger signals) from the muscles reaches a threshold, at which point pain suddenly appears.

Basically, trigger points activate nociception receptors, which sensitize the CNS, and the CNS responds with the sensation of pain in a different part of the body. And because of the brain's ability to change—the more often this phenomenon occurs, the more likely the CNS will "stick" in this pattern. With this under-standing, we, as bodyworkers, can unstick the body to help the brain revert to being pain-free.

I'll go deeper into the details of direct and satellite pain referral in Chapter 6.

How Do Trigger Points Develop?

There is a general consensus now that trigger points develop when the demands on muscle fibers exceed their metabolic capacity.

As an example, in the conduct of war, you must preserve and protect supply chains. If you can't feed your soldiers, they will wear out and become ineffective. Muscles are no different. They require

---

24 A significant portion of their research involved injecting muscle areas with saline and recording what pain pattern was reported. The saline injection causes a temporary inflammatory response where the trigger points would normally develop (behind the shoulder in the case of infraspinatus), and the reported pain mimics the referral.

food in the form of energy molecules, or they become unable to do the basic work of contraction.

Muscles also require toxic metabolic waste products to be transported out of the cells regularly. Bringing nutrients in and waste products out happens in the finest filaments of the vascular system, the capillaries. When the surrounding tissues become inflamed, these delicate vessels can easily become blocked and ineffective.

Athletes train by placing incremental demands on their muscles, and as they ramp up the demand, their bodies develop more muscle and more efficient vascularization. In other words, they have more developed capillary networks with more redundancy and can deliver nutrients under more extreme conditions than the average couch potato. A properly trained athlete can overload their muscles temporarily and not have lasting effects other than some soreness. Their highly developed vascular systems can overcome the temporary local stresses and inflammatory response in their tissues, and their muscles can quickly repair and transport toxins out.

Trigger points can be *active* or *latent*. Active trigger points are what cause a clinical complaint. Latent trigger points don't cause a perceptible sensation but may be causing postural changes and other subliminal effects. At any time, latent trigger points can rise above a threshold and become active. This is very confusing, as pain comes and goes, seemingly unrelated to whatever diagnosis the patient has been assigned. Latent does not mean less important. In my experience, latent effects can be profound and a significant factor in satellite referral chains.

Acute versus Chronic Overload

When the CNS demands work from a muscle, the muscle must be able to contract with enough force to overcome the resistance without running out of fuel, meaning the energy provided by nutrients such as ATP. Overload can be acute or chronic. *Acute overload* happens when the momentary demands on a muscle are more than the muscle can deliver. The capillaries—the smallest blood vessels in the body—are a key player in this process, delivering nutrients to the muscles as well as flushing out waste. If the flow of nutrients is inadequate, inflammatory substances may develop at the cellular level, and the capillaries won't be able to flush them out. Edema—a build-up of excess fluid—can constrict the ability of the capillaries even further, so a vicious cycle occurs.

Trigger points from acute overload can be relatively easy to analyze and treat if only local muscles are involved. We can take a look at the pain pattern, the description of the event, and surmise which muscle was affected. In relatively few situations, the issue might involve a muscle or two rather than an entire system. In these cases, trigger point therapy works well and seems miraculous; you treat one or two muscles, and the pain quickly goes away. However, these cases are rare. Even with acute overload, satellite referral can set up the local muscle to be more vulnerable to disturbance, in which case treating that muscle won't produce lasting results.

Chronic overload is more ubiquitous, more subtle, harder to analyze, and generally involves wider patterns of muscles. In addition, the brain becomes upregulated to some extent, so we have to also reset the nervous system to a normal level of sensitivity. As pain goes on for hours and days, the CNS becomes increasingly sensitized, recruiting additional muscles to provide stability and protect against further injury—whether or not it occurs. We see this quite often in the case of what mainstream medicine calls frozen shoulder syndrome. In our analysis, we must look at the biomechanical event that took place, try to understand which muscles were stressed, and determine if they could be transmitting their dysfunction through a chain of muscles, ending with the ones causing the immediate pain.

Postural muscles, such as the lower trapezius, are particularly vulnerable to chronic overload. The body recruits smaller postural stabilization fibers first when having to stabilize posture during repetitive tasks.[25] These fibers are activated first and deactivated last, and they are also the smallest, which sets them up for overload. If we don't have balanced posture, the load on these stabilizer fibers can increase dramatically. In addition, they're relatively small, so they don't have the robust ability to ramp up their capacity that strength-oriented muscles (such as the pectoralis major or quadriceps) do.

When acute pain develops due to sudden overuse—for example, unusual sports activities or bracing for a fall off a bike or slipping on ice—conventional medical professionals will invariably assume that an injury was involved. However, trigger points resulting from temporary muscle overload can produce pain as compelling and dramatic as an injury, and in my experience, this is by far the most common cause. Pain that persists after six to eight weeks is no longer related to soft tissue damage because the body repairs damaged tissues within that time.

---

25 Shah et al., "Myofascial Trigger Points Then and Now," 6.

"Joe is an avid cross country skier and had almost given up on skate skiing because of pain in his right knee caused during the season three years ago. The pain presented on the lateral aspect of the knee, alongside the knee cap. I noticed the right foot showed more signs of pronation than the left. This was apparent in the foot calluses and the wear on the bottom of the shoes showing a pattern of bracing. Since I was trained in the lower body protocol, the treatment began at the source muscle, the QL, and continued to a treatment of all gluteus muscles, with a focus on gluteus minimus, which referred to the vastus lateralis. Upper leg treatment included vastus lateralis and the adductors as antagonists, followed by the full stretches of these areas. The results were astounding.

"Joe has resumed his skiing in both classic and skate skiing with no pain since the session. He also commented that he now has no pain while climbing stairs—the first time in years!"

—Krista Matison, CTB advanced practitioner,
Grand Rapids, Minnesota

CHAPTER 5

How Muscles Misbehave

When muscles develop trigger points, they can misbehave in a variety of uncomfortable, painful, and disruptive ways. Unless practitioners understand that these patterns of dysfunction are commonly caused by trigger points rather than injury or disease, they are likely to pursue inappropriate treatments that make the situation worse.

Strength Deficits

Many patients come to our clinic having been assessed by a physical therapist or other medical professional as having a "strength deficit." In these cases, the patient has failed a strength machine evaluation, and the doctor will assign them strengthening exercises for whichever muscles tested weak. But often, these muscles aren't truly weak at all; they have developed trigger points that lead to dysfunction. The strengthening exercises, prescribed by a doctor or therapist who doesn't understand trigger points, can make the pain worse rather than relieving it because trigger points are easily created in situations involving acute overload.

Remember that once a muscle becomes overloaded and develops trigger points, some percentage of its fibers are essentially taken offline and locked in a contracture; they become taut fibers. When a motor signal is sent to the muscle, many of its fibers cannot respond because they are already contracted. These taut fibers send danger signals to the spinal cord, which can cause active pain referral. As a result, when the patient tries to engage the muscle, they are likely to feel pain as the muscle bunches up. In addition, once the CNS receives those danger signals during a muscular contraction, it can inhibit that muscle and engage its antagonist as a way to provide safety. So inevitably, the muscle isn't going to look good on a strength test.

When we look at these "strength deficits" through the lens of trigger point therapy, we can see that resistance training for strength is inappropriate in the early phases of treatment. Before we can ask the muscle to take on more work, we have to help the muscle fibers become healthy. Otherwise, if you put additional demands with resistance training on muscles that have trigger points, that's a formula for more overload, and they are likely to get worse. This happens often and is a primary cause of failed therapy.[26]

Resistance to Stretch

Another sign that trigger points are present in a muscle or muscular system is limited or compromised range of motion in the corresponding joint or joints. This phenomenon is often present in so-called frozen shoulder syndrome.

Resistance to stretch is an easy phenomenon to reproduce in a muscle with trigger points. As the muscle lengthens, the taut fibers attempt to lengthen as well, pulling apart the area of the sarcomeres in contracture. This mechanical disturbance of the

---

26 This is not to say that strength is a bad thing. Athletes can tolerate much higher levels of insult to their muscles because they train and have vascular and strength reserves. They are much more likely to self-repair trigger points than someone without those reserves. In the CTB system, balanced strength and flexibility is an important goal that we pursue after the initial phases of treatment.

trigger point will tend to irritate the contracted tissues and stimulate the nociceptive compounds in the trigger point, increasing their signaling to the spinal cord. Discomfort will increase, and the patient may notice pain in the stretching fibers as well as the referral zone of the muscle. The pain may ramp up dramatically, and at that point it becomes too uncomfortable to push farther into the stretch without applying some means of distraction, such as therapeutic vibration. As soon as there is a pain response, the CNS tends to go into protective mode by locking things down with muscular engagement. For the CNS, reduced motion equals increased stability and safety, and taut fibers from trigger points are a useful way to provide additional stability without excessive energy demands.

Stretching a muscle with trigger points is a reliable way to produce its pain referral pattern and assess which muscles are responsible for a pain pattern. It is not, however, a good first step in treatment. In cases where range of motion is limited and the muscles are resistant to stretch, it's a mistake to try to lengthen muscles before therapeutic and rehabilitative work on the tissues. Stretching must be done incrementally, and there are various hacks that we can use to prevent the CNS from embedding more trigger points to protect against injury, which we'll go into later.

Grabbing, Shaking, Twitching

The amount that a muscle can lengthen without distress (its stretch range) is an important criterion, but its *quality of motion* is equally important. A patient might be able to move their joint into a range that seems normal; hypermobile individuals might be able to move into a range that exceeds normal.

If trigger points are present in the muscle or its antagonist, you may notice that the muscle periodically "grabs," resisting lengthening or shortening. You must move the joint slowly, paying close attention, or you might miss it. You might also notice a muscle twitching at rest or feeling shaky and unstable when the client attempts to engage it. This is a strong sign that taut fibers are sending disturbing signals to the spinal cord, confusing the system about how to respond.

Muscle spasms may accompany trigger point dysfunction. Some muscles spasm when you try to shorten their fibers if they have embedded taut fibers. You may have experienced this phenomenon in the form of a charley horse in the hamstrings or calves. Once the spasm starts, you basically have to wait until it subsides. They aren't necessarily painful, but they compromise the muscle's ability to both lengthen and shorten. We will cover the topic of shortening dysfunction in detail in a later section.

When an aircraft is gaining speed for takeoff, the pilots are paying close attention to how the engines are responding so they can catch any issues before pushing the throttle and leaving the ground. Similarly, the CNS receives constant feedback from both sides of the joint as we move. If disturbing signals are coming in as you move a joint, the CNS may quickly vacillate between engagement and release, and smooth motion may be impossible.

Poor Balance and Coordination

Poor balance might also be an indicator that trigger points have developed in the body. Good balance, as in standing on one foot, requires a constant, fluid interplay between muscles on both sides of a joint. Balance poses such as tree pose in yoga aren't static experiences—the muscles controlling the ankle and foot must perform continual micro-corrections to maintain stability. If these movements become too large, the person will wobble and shake.

Trigger points can negatively affect one's balance and coordination by sending erroneous signals to the CNS regarding muscle tension and length. This process can disturb the coordination between agonist and antagonist muscles, resulting in poor balance. Related signs include dropping things, poor fine motor control, reduced ability to play musical instruments, poor performance in sports, and similar problems.

Muscle Inhibition

The manual therapy field has a concept called *muscle inhibition* that is based on the observation that muscles sometimes don't engage when or as fully as they should. It can also describe a situation when muscles that should contract simultaneously fire in succession, causing imbalance in the joints and even in the position of bones. While the concept is well established, there has been no suitable explanation for why it occurs.

To better understand this phenomenon, let's look at a prime example. A muscle that commonly becomes inhibited is vastus medialis, the medial short quadricep head. Proper coordination of the four heads of the quadriceps muscles is critical to ensuring that the kneecap (patella) moves in the proper direction and doesn't rub against its track, potentially causing a condition known as chondromalacia patella. Chondromalacia describes damage to the patella that can occur if it consistently rubs against a side wall of its track.

The quadriceps have oblique attachments to the tendon that controls the kneecap. The branch on the outside of the leg (vastus lateralis) is a larger, more powerful muscle than the inside quadricep (vastus medialis). Each muscle can pull the patella toward itself; ideally, both pulling at once will keep the patella centered as the knee extends.

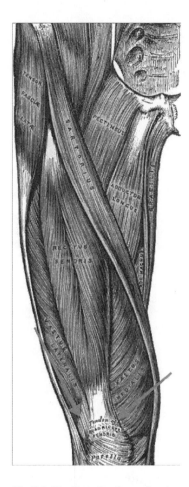

Fig. 5-1. The fiber directions of vastus medialis and vastus lateralis should result in a balanced pull on the patella, keeping it centered in its track. Colorized by Michael Gasperl, *Gray's Anatomy*, Public Domain, https://commons.wikimedia.org/w/index.php?curid=31906481.

When a patient develops pain and swelling around the knee, it is common to observe that the vastus medialis doesn't contract right away as the patient tries to extend their knee, causing the patella to immediately divert in a lateral direction. This is sometimes called inhibition of the vastus medialis, or it may be identified as a "firing order problem." Because the vastus lateralis contracts first, it pulls the patella more strongly in the lateral direction, causing the patella to rub on the outside of its track and generating inflammation, possibly even damaging the bone surface.

In the case of an inhibited vastus medialis, the patient will likely feel pain around their knee, but the root cause is often trigger points in other, more distant muscles. In some cases the body seems to let one side of a functional antagonist relationship dominate when dysfunction develops. We have had great success eliminating the inhibition phenomenon by applying our CTB protocols, which consider muscles on both sides of the joint as well as all satellite referral sources.

Shortening Dysfunction and How It Blocks Stretch

Healthy muscles can be stretched or shortened without causing pain or other discomfort. Most people are familiar with stretching and know that certain muscles will feel uncomfortable if you attempt to stretch them beyond a certain point. Very few people realize that muscles can become dysfunctional when shortened. In fact, *shortening dysfunction* is an even more significant issue than stretching dysfunction and can occur with either passive or active shortening.

Active shortening occurs when you engage a muscle. If you use your biceps and brachialis to bend your elbow, those muscles are contracting actively and the overall length of the fibers becomes shorter than they were with the elbow straight. If you rest your arm in a bent position, such as during sleep, you are no longer actively contracting those muscles. At that point we say that biceps and brachialis are being passively shortened.

Normally, muscles become softer when in passive shortening, so a telltale sign of shortening dysfunction is the muscle hardening as it is shortened. This indicates that a type of automatic spasm or contraction is happening within the muscle without a motor signal from the spine telling the fibers to engage. This condition can sometimes be painful, and even if not, it can stop the joint from bending any further, meaning that it inhibits the stretch of the muscle's antagonists.

For example, a patient might describe pain in their adductors (inner thigh) muscles when you put those muscles on stretch. They might feel tension or discomfort in the adductors but not realize that the gluteus muscles are quietly limiting the adductor stretch from the other side of the hip joint. These gluteal fibers might not produce any pain during the adductor stretch (though they often do), but if you palpate them you will find that instead of softening as they passively shorten, they harden. If you manage to lengthen the adductors sufficiently and ask the client what they're feeling, they might report cramping or pain or even what they call "stretching" in the hardened, bunched up gluteal fibers at the end of the adductor stretch. This is due to shortening dysfunction.

"After her surgery for ectopic pregnancy, Libby started to have severe cramps with menstruation each month and stabbing/sharp pain in the right side of her lower abdomen and pelvis that radiated into an aching, constant discomfort in the side flank/back. After seeing countless practitioners, her doctor diagnosed her with endometriosis because they did not know where else to attribute the pain. The doctor thought the surgery 'triggered' endometriosis and made it worse/apparent, which she had never had symptoms of prior to surgery. The piece that was fishy to me was that her menstrual cycles were not heavy at all; she in fact had light bleeding each month. This doesn't add up with endometriosis, which usually involves severe bleeding.

"During evaluation, I discovered that Libby is a severe hyperpronator and is on her feet all day long as a nurse. She also has some anxiety/stress issues and I discovered she is a dysfunctional breather.

"In our first session, we found her low obliques and low rectus abdominis were involved in her abdominal pain. Her psoas major and iliacus created direct referral into what she called her 'flank pain.' Her right QL/iliocostalis were directly related to her back pain. She has a postural collapse from the ankles up due to hyperpronation, and her QLs are very taut.

"We ordered her hyperpronation correction inserts and met again after her next menstrual cycle to see how things felt during the time when her pain would normally be most expressed. She came back and reported NO pain since our first session and that her menstrual cycle was very easy with no discomfort. She had also had no back pain. During our second session, we fit her into inserts and worked with her adductors and revisited the abdominal and back muscles from first session.

"Libby has been living pain free, her periods are no longer extremely painful, and she is so relieved that her issues are not
organ related or endometriosis. She had thought for years since
the surgery that she might not be able to have children and would
need to do exploratory surgery for endometriosis and might have
lifelong pain and dysfunction."

—Jill Duncan, CTB master practitioner,
St. Louis, Missouri

CHAPTER 6

Upgrading from Trigger Point 1.0 to 2.0

While I truly feel that the trigger point work of Travell and Simons is one of the great, if undervalued, achievements of modern medicine, I have found the original manifestation of their work to have practical limitations. Travell brought these phenomena out of obscurity and presented them to her medical colleagues, who remained her primary audience for many years. Today, there are a select few expert trigger point therapists who have independently found a way to expand these ideas and make them more practical and reliable. Few MDs still incorporate it into their practice. To broaden the reach and effectiveness of these ideas, I would like to propose some updates based on current neuroscience along with my last fifteen years of clinical experience.

As I attempted to apply concepts from Travell and Simons (and later, Davies) to my own developing CTB modality, I had significant success with my clients but also many failures to relieve them of their pain. It took me some years to understand that my failures were an inevitable result of some limitations in the way these ideas were expressed in the original books as well as the medical world into which they were born.

The idea that you press a magic button (the trigger point) and pain will go away is an unfortunate oversimplification of the theory. The trigger point is viewed as the enemy, and if we overpower it, it will stop referring pain, and our problems will be solved. In this interpretation, the trigger point is treated as the pathology. If we get rid of the "bad guy," the pain will go away, not unlike surgery on an injury.

However, I see the trigger point itself as a symptom, not a cause, and in many cases, trigger points are there to help the body maintain structure and stability. I don't see them as an unfortunate mistake; rather, they are aligned with the body's protective attempts to compensate for problematic circumstances. I see my role as getting inside the body's compensatory logic to help me understand how to move past the stopgap measures to a higher state of harmony and balance—and less pain.

While she was recognized as a brilliant researcher, Travell's work never received widespread adoption, even in the medical community. Travell and Simons focused on two primary modalities for treating trigger points: (1) injection with procaine, a local anesthetic, and (2) a technique known as "spray and stretch."

Injection, the Original Trigger Point Treatment Modality

Dr. Travell's primary treatment approach was injecting trigger points with procaine, a local anesthetic. The needle mechanically disrupts the trigger point and breaks up stagnation so metabolic exchange can resume. The procaine has no effect on the trigger point and is necessary to minimize inflammation and pain from the needle itself; needles for injection are much larger and damage more tissue than acupuncture needles.

While the injection approach can be effective, it presents numerous challenges in terms of adoption and the likelihood of success. The greatest hurdle for injection is that only those medical professionals with a license to inject can practice the technique. And even for them, they can face daunting issues.

For one, trigger point injection requires a highly detailed under-standing of musculoskeletal anatomy, something which few MDs have outside of their area of specialty. Foot and ankle surgeons understand that area of the body extremely well but would be lost in other parts of the body. Trigger point injection requires practitioners to have precise knowledge of the location of nerves and blood vessels. Practitioners must also know which areas are vulnerable to harm if punctured. They must identify and isolate taut fibers, which requires muscular palpation skills that typical medical training might not include.

Secondly, muscles cannot be moved while the needle is inserted, making it impossible to guide muscles through range during treat-ment, which I have found to be essential for retraining the CNS.

Thirdly, there is a practical limit to how many sites can be injected in a sitting. Injection needles are roughly a hundred times thicker than acupuncture needles and do cause tissue damage and pain. Injection lends itself most readily to isolated activations in one or two muscles, which is a fairly rare scenario.

Another major obstacle in the way of the injection approach is the time required to administer it. Any nontrivial trigger point case takes time for analysis, testing, and setup for injections, followed by integrating movements. But the care model in the United States makes it nearly impossible for physicians to spend any more than fifteen minutes with a patient, so the hour or more required to administer injections is not feasible.

The most enthusiastic audience for Travell's ideas, in the be-ginning, were dentists and orthodontists. They already knew the relevant anatomy of the head and neck, were comfortable injecting local anesthetics in regional structures, and were used to dealing with relatively small muscles whose fibers were easy to understand. Dentists also have a significant incentive to avoid unnecessary extractions, and trigger points are a well-known source of intense tooth and jaw pain. That being said, even in dental programs, trigger point knowledge is rare.

While Travell intended her work primarily for MDs, the medical community was not well suited for either adoption or practical success. Manual therapists would have been a more suitable audience, but manual techniques were not in the purview of the original textbooks.

Spray and Stretch: Using Distraction

The other primary modality covered in the medical texts is known as spray and stretch. A practitioner sprays a very focused stream of intense coolant on a trigger point to shock and distract the nervous system, masking the usual pain referral patterns as muscles are stretched. Travell and Simons used spray and stretch because they needed something less focal and specific than injection. They recognized the need to move muscles within and beyond their range of motion following injection for the CNS to integrate the treatment and to prevent the issues from returning.

During a spray and stretch treatment, the therapist must have access to both the trigger point area in the offending muscle(s) and also the referral zones. They must apply it directly to the skin in a thin stream while moving the muscle to and through its stretch barrier. The therapist moves the spray slowly, so it covers the trigger point and referral zones.

Spray and stretch takes advantage of a neurological phenomenon known as distraction. The cold thin line of spray is such a dramatic input to the nervous system that it overwhelms the danger signals from the tissues and the patient's perception of pain that would normally become evident as the muscle is stretched. Without pain during stretch, the body can let the taut fibers lengthen without protective engagement of the muscle due to the stretch response, which is a natural tendency of the body to engage fibers to control stretch. It works quite well with some muscles.

It is important to note that the benefits afforded by this technique have nothing to do with cooling the muscle. In fact, to the extent that the fibers are cooled, they will become more resistant to treatment because, at their core, trigger points are areas of microcellular metabolic stagnation. Cooling tissues decreases metabolic exchange, which is the last thing we want. During a spray and stretch session, the therapist uses a heat source to rewarm tissues after spraying.

In spite of its practical limitations, this modality works quite well because it takes advantage of how the CNS can be "rewired" through distraction. Spray and stretch defeats the CNS's protective response when pain is produced during the stretch. But, like injection, the technique has quite a few pitfalls.

Travell first tried ethyl chloride, which also happened to be a powerful and highly flammable general anesthetic. Spraying in an enclosed space was dangerous and led to some unfortunate events, including some doctors losing consciousness and falling, presenting unacceptable risks for both doctor and patient. The replacement product, Fluori-Methane, was found to be bad for the ozone layer. The current product, still manufactured by Gebauer & Co., is inert, without psychoactive effects, but is expensive and expendable, making it undesirable for frequent therapeutic use.

Another limitation is that the spray must be applied to bare skin. Positions must be carefully planned so the therapist can spray both the trigger point zone and the referral zone while moving the muscle into stretch. This is often impossible without assistance from another therapist or practitioner.

Even with its limitations and toxicity, that spray and stretch works so well is a testament to the neurological basis for trigger points, which has heavily informed my Coaching the Body ideas.

Approaches to Manual Therapy

The Travell and Simons materials made passing reference to the use of manual therapy, but it wasn't their area of expertise. Clair Davies's biggest contribution, in his own view, was using his background as a skilled piano mechanic to come up with manual therapy techniques for each muscle. He was accustomed to detail work with technology and sticking with a problem until it was solved. He was able to wade through the highly technical Travell and Simons books on his own and translate their ideas into useful manual therapy techniques.

Even though his work was a huge advance, I found certain things to be absent. Davies wasn't a fan of movement or stretching. His primary technique involves cross-fiber compression without change of fiber length or any kind of resolving stretches. That said, he was very interested in my experiments bringing Thai techniques to trigger point work, but he had no background in Thai techniques himself.

The teaching of trigger point therapy in massage schools has been flawed (if it's even included in the curriculum). At most, it's usually a bullet point in an alternative modality lecture. Over half of my students are already massage therapists, and for the most part, they come in with rudimentary or nonexistent trigger point knowledge. Without any coverage from the originators of trigger point theory, it's understandable that manual therapy has remained in the dark ages as an implementation vehicle for the theory.

CROSS-FIBER COMPRESSION

Clair Davies provided an important contribution for manual therapists, but his *cross-fiber compression* technique is still only partially successful. Like ischemic compression, it fails to provide an experience of integrative movement to the CNS. Clair's approach was to find a taut fiber and use the thumbs or a tool to stroke across the fiber direction twelve times and then move on. There was no joint movement or stretching of the muscle involved. He felt that natural everyday movements would eventually integrate the changes in the tissues.

ISCHEMIC COMPRESSION

Davies's cross-fiber techniques were somewhat of an improvement over what is generally taught to massage therapists. The translation of trigger points into massage school curricula, when it's even taught, generally involves using a simpler technique called *ischemic compression*. The therapist finds a tender point, compresses it, voiding fluids from the local area, and waits twelve seconds or so for the muscle to "release." When pressure is released, fluids return, and with them, some additional level of metabolic exchange, allowing the cell to clear inflammatory compounds and bring in essential substances to provide energy to the cell. While it can assist in disrupting the trigger points, ischemic compression is inadequate as a sole means of addressing trigger point-related issues. Each muscle has its own architecture, fiber arrangements, and characteristics. One technique doesn't fit all.

Simple ischemic compression produces pain and uses no distraction, and the lack of movement greatly impedes any ability to retrain the CNS. Compressing the point will likely invoke local tenderness and pain referral if there is no attempt at distraction. In response, the CNS will perpetuate muscular engagement to protect the area. Without movement, we cannot adequately exploit the brain's innate ability to downregulate and desensitize the CNS. Joint movement engages the neurological relationships between agonist and antagonist muscle groups and is how we can quickly help the CNS regain the capacity for pain-free movement. Having the client suffer through undistracted pain referral is likely to cause the CNS to upregulate and make things worse and further restrict range of motion rather than allowing more.

Reliance upon compression without movement, along with a lack of understanding of muscle relationships, has caused manual therapists to relegate trigger point therapy to their large collection of techniques that work occasionally but don't deserve the spotlight. They weren't trained in a way that set them up for success.

For example, many clients have hard, tender fibers in their high trapezius, and therapists often lay into the hard muscle with elbows. This is a bad approach for many reasons. First of all, the real issues are likely not even in the high trapezius but in muscles that refer into it as a satellite (such as low trapezius fibers and serratus anterior). The high trapezius is a stress-sensitive muscle, part of the body's innate protective response. The so-called "fighter's reflex" consists of elevating the shoulders with high trapezius fibers to protect the sensitive areas of the neck. Causing undistracted pain in this muscle without any movement is likely to increase danger signals to the CNS, leaving the client with sore shoulders, a headache, and no relief.

The Direct Referral Trap

Direct referral is generally how most people first understand trigger point therapy. I use the term *direct referral* for the pain pattern of a single muscle. Travell and Simons spent decades identifying the core concepts and documenting the direct referral patterns and behavior for over a hundred muscles, along with the anatomy, functional and neurological characteristics, and much more—an enormous achievement. It remains a monumental effort, but it's incomplete.

The first time you see a pain referral chart, it can be a heady and even exciting experience. The secrets of the universe appear to be laid out in front of you. It's easy to fall in love with the idea that every pain has a magic release point, and if you work on that point, you can make the pain go away.

I certainly felt that way when I first opened Clair Davies's *Trigger Point Workbook*, examining its maps of tender points and where they produced pain. At that time, I had only been at my Thai massage practice for a few years, and while I knew that pain often had nonlocal origins, I couldn't find any sort of map that associated pain patterns with source points. So, of course, I immediately went out and tried it on myself and everyone I could get my hands on. I found that I could often reproduce aspects of the pain pattern by compressing a muscle's trigger points, but actually finding the points could be challenging, and often the pain would go away temporarily but then return. Sometimes it would get worse. Something else was at play beyond direct referral.

After years of clinical experience, I now know that direct referral can be a trap.

It is very tempting to look at a referral chart and jump to the offending muscle, finding and treating the one trigger point that is most likely to be referring the pain. Without much training, a trigger point therapist is likely to make a list of candidate muscles based on the Travell and Simons priority list for a given pain area, and they'll design their approach by working down the list without being aware that the muscles are interdependent, related neurologically, and should be treated in a specific order.

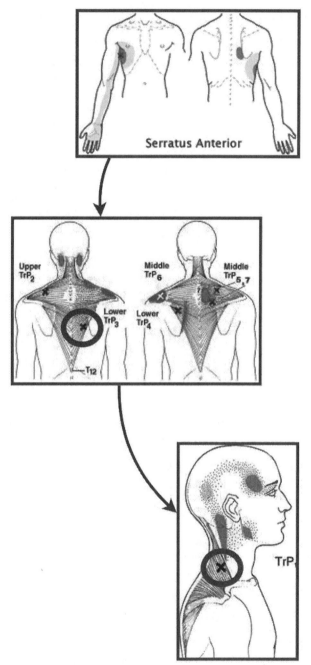

Fig. 6-1. Satellite referral from the serratus anterior to the low trapezius to the high trapezius, resulting in headache pain.

Satellite referral, on the other hand, is a chain that develops when one muscle's direct referral pattern lands geographically over another muscle's trigger point areas and causes dysfunction of some sort in the second muscle.

Muscles don't just randomly become dysfunctional. They respond to inputs in the body from other muscles, biomechanics, postural asymmetry, and much more. Even when working with a fairly specific pain pattern, it is highly unlikely that only a single muscle is responsible. The muscle that speaks the loudest is most likely the one at the end of a chain. But other muscles contribute, even if they aren't reflected in a visible pain pattern. The muscle at the end of the chain is being set up by other muscles, and unless you treat these chains at the source, the results will be disappointing.

Because it ignores the sophisticated neuromuscular relationships in the body, the single muscle direct referral approach is doomed—if not to failure, then to mediocrity. Either it doesn't work at all, or the pain fades but returns. Some people are perfectly happy alleviating pain for a few hours or days, but I was never satisfied with that.

In twenty years of developing my approach, the most important work I have done is uncovering these hidden relationships that are secret progenitors of pain and organizing them into treatment protocols.

Understanding the True Importance of Satellite Referral

Travell and Simons recognized that there was more at work than a simple direct referral relationship, and they even mentioned satellite referral several times in their books, but their research in this area was spotty, and the descriptions are incomplete and not fully fleshed out. The concept remained a bit of an afterthought, and editors of the third edition have reduced its importance even more, lumping it in with other "associated trigger points" and relegating it to background material as part of consolidating all the work into a single volume. Even the original editions don't discuss many of the common satellite patterns that we observe every day in my school.

I find that this obscures what we have seen clinically to be an extremely important mechanism. The physiological mechanism behind referral is still very much a subject of active research. Even though we don't have a solid explanation for how referral happens, the fact that it does is indisputable to anyone with a rudimentary level of experience with trigger point therapy.

So, if the medical world has trouble understanding direct referral, satellite referral is even stranger. The idea that one muscle can produce a kind of phantom pain and then that pain can cause another muscle to develop problems is a bit tough to swallow for hard science advocates.

The phenomenon of satellite referral consists of the referral pattern of one muscle (the key) disturbing the proprioceptive field of another (the satellite). For example, Muscle A may have a referral pattern that lies over Muscle B's trigger point area. In response to this disturbance, Muscle B may itself develop a trigger point. Any muscle whose referral pattern falls over another may cause the satellite to develop trigger points in response. This chain may then continue for several more muscles. The client may only report the pain from the satellite muscle at the end of the chain—a very common circumstance. Essentially, this sets up a hidden network that cannot be detected on its own without a reference catalogue of satellite referral paths. Unless you already know the likely path these referrals can take, they are very difficult to discern via observation.

In my research, I've encountered widespread, recurring satellite patterns that occur very frequently, many of which were not mentioned in Travell and Simons. Travell and Simons suggested that only active trigger points can produce dysfunction in other muscles. However, I have seen many cases in which the client had no experience of direct referral from certain muscles but did experience profound satellite referral effects, sometimes several steps away from the originating muscle.

It has become clear to me via years of clinical observation that satellite referral is very real and can operate in a kind of shadow network beneath the observed surface phenomena, even if many of the steps are latent. It's a safe bet to assume that satellite effects are operative in most common pain patterns. In our clinical work over the last two decades, we've found satellite referral to be far more important and profound than we could have imagined, and it is now a core principle of the CTB system.

THE IMPORTANCE OF FUNCTIONAL RELATIONSHIPS

The body rarely uses a single muscle to accomplish a task. Muscles have certain actions in common and others that are opposed. Having two muscles pulling in opposite directions is necessary for stability. In a tug of war, if one side suddenly lets go, the forces are no longer balanced, and the other side will probably fall over. For example, we have four individual quadriceps muscles, and they all collaborate to extend the knee. Within this collaboration, the inner quad (vastus medialis) and the outer quad (vastus lateralis) move the patella in opposite directions due to their position and fiber direction.

Because of this need for stability, the CNS is constantly monitoring muscles that are in functional opposition as a unit. If one side becomes taut and shortened, the other side will likely develop trigger points as well. Trigger points, as we have covered elsewhere in this book, are useful as a means of adding stability to a joint without the demands of constant muscular engagement.

What this implies is that we generally cannot resolve issues on one side of a functional relationship without including the functional antagonist(s) in our work as well. Often, the fastest way to get a muscle to release its taut fibers is through therapeutic work on its antagonist. Then when we return to the original muscle, we find that it's much easier to get it to release. This approach permeates CTB protocols. When you closely examine the organization of modules within each protocol, they generally treat functional antagonists together or in close proximity. When we change a muscle's length during therapy, we often provide feedback in the form of manual compression on its antagonists.

Thai Massage for Pain: The Good and the Bad

Thai massage, the bodywork form that I initially trained in and practiced for many years, involves a lot of movement and complex interactions that influence more than one muscle at a time. These techniques evolved in the context of the traditional Thai medical system, which is built on a completely different set of concepts than Western anatomy-based systems. In fact, there is no concept of muscles in traditional Thai medicine. The techniques of Thai massage are powerful tools that are often used indiscriminately, with no awareness of functional anatomy, and can produce negative results because of an excessive focus on vigorous stretches and painful compression. That being said, after some years of experimentation, I found that if you understand their muscular effects, some Thai bodywork techniques add a powerful dimension to trigger point therapy precisely because these techniques can integrate work in multiple systems at once, are often movement-based, and provide distraction by overwhelming the CNS with input.

Traditional Thai massage training—like what I studied—does not consider the muscular effects of the poses, and therefore there are no manuals or books with that kind of information. I spent years cata-loguing the techniques I had learned along with an analysis of their effects on the muscular system. Fortunately, through my in-depth study of Travell and Simons, I gained a comprehensive knowledge of functional anatomy as it relates to trigger point therapy and was able to adapt and sequence Thai techniques in an appropriate way. In my teaching, I am careful to inform my students of the muscular effects of any included Thai techniques, so they can have their own framework for understanding what makes sense and in what order.

In their traditional setting, many of the Thai techniques are performed in a sequence that makes no sense for a pain client. For example, muscles are often vigorously stretched with no preparatory manual compression, which is asking for disaster in a muscle loaded with trigger points, particularly in a client not used to stretching. We have to understand that Thai massage developed in a culture much different from that of the United States. In general, people are more active, they don't tend to sit in chairs at desk jobs, and are, on the whole, far more fluid and flexible than typical Westerners. There also tends to be a "no pain, no gain" mentality among some Thai practitioners, which ignores the protective role of the CNS and, in the hands of the wrong practitioner, can leave the client in a worse state than they began.

With my knowledge of both trigger point therapy and Thai massage, I started to develop my own approach with the aim of integrating modern medical understanding of muscular function and the role of the CNS in the pain response with the traditional movement-based modality of Thai massage.

MODIFYING THAI TECHNIQUES TO "HACK" THE CNS

When I started applying Thai techniques to trigger point work, I used some elements of the traditional practice while leaving out others. I designed techniques that allow the therapist to interact with muscles on both sides of the joint simultaneously. For example, rather than treating the tibialis anterior in the shin first (running into limitations from the compromised soleus on the other side of the ankle joint), CTB includes a technique based on Thai bodywork that allows the therapist to move the ankle into dorsiflexion and plantar flexion while providing compressive feedback to both of those muscles at once.

As I've mentioned before, muscles are not autonomous, and they don't work in isolation. Not only do they work in concert with other muscles, they are also controlled by the CNS, which gathers proprioceptive signals from the muscle as well as its functional agonists and antagonists, determining how the system will behave. Trigger points are messengers reporting to the CNS via nociception that something is wrong in the local milieu of the muscle. That report does not equate to pain or limitation; it is simply nociceptive information, which the brain then decides how to interpret.

In order to create a modality that would treat not only the trigger muscle but also its system, with the aim of downregulating and "hacking" the CNS, I have designed techniques that allow the therapist to interact with muscles on both sides of the joint simultaneously. Instead of focusing primarily on resolving one muscle at a time, this approach recognizes that the conductor of the orchestra—the CNS—monitors and also determines the condition of the players in both functional units, and they must be treated as a system. Neuroplastic change in the nervous system causes and allows fast change in the taut fibers in the opposing muscles.

Consequently, in the CTB system, we use techniques that allow us to influence both sides of the joint simultaneously without having to change positions. This difference in approach has a dramatic practical effect. Change happens more quickly, and it is more sustainable because we're downregulating the CNS. In some cases, the Thai technique repertoire naturally incorporates the concept of working both sides of the joint. In others, we had to adapt the original technique. Overall, these techniques provide a rich framework if the therapist is armed with the correct knowledge.

WORKING ON THE FLOOR VERSUS THE TABLE

Thai massage has been historically practiced with the client on floor mats, which generally allows the therapist to use body weight more effectively. Some Western therapists initially see working on the floor as a barrier due to their own limitations in flexibility or simply the fact that their current setup is built around a table. In my own practice, I have always had and used both. Each has benefits, and most of the Thai techniques can be easily adapted to the table. Certain techniques actually benefit from room to stand and the leverage of the legs pushing off the floor. You can practice CTB very effectively on the table or on a mat.

Adapting the techniques to the table may involve placing one or both hips on the table, which makes a table wider than thirty inches best. The working weight of the table should be at least 500 pounds, and any kind of variable height control such as a hydraulic mechanism is a nice but unnecessary feature. I've recorded several videos on the topic of doing CTB on the table; scan the QR code for an explanatory video with some examples.

Fig. 6-2. Table work QR code.

Satellite Referral in Practice:
Shoulder Pain

Shoulder pain is quite common and often created by dysfunction in the infraspinatus muscle and its anterior shoulder referral pattern in the front of the body. A new bodyworker might be tempted to focus primarily on this muscle at the beginning of a treatment, but time is better spent addressing the system of muscles involved in and around the shoulder girdle that could be setting this muscle up for dysfunction.

Every massage student learns that the primary action of the infraspinatus is external rotation of the humerus (upper arm bone). However, we need to look at its functional role in the shoulder, not just its external rotation action, in order to fully understand its vulnerabilities. The infraspinatus is a critical stabilizer during any movement of the humerus. The shoulder is a highly mobile joint, and in order to avoid injury, the muscles of the rotator cuff must collaborate to stabilize the arm in the glenoid fossa (shoulder socket). If the head of the humerus was to move without careful control and stability, it would erratically impinge upon the connective tissue within the joint, causing injury and disease.

Anyone with severe shoulder pain is likely to exhibit an anterior pain pattern during arm motion. An inexperienced therapist might notice this pain and attempt to treat the infraspinatus, so the referral stops. What they are likely to find is that the muscle is very resistant to treatment. In our CTB Upper Body Protocol, we defer treatment of infraspinatus until the scapular positioning and rotation muscles have been thoroughly treated.

Functionally, all of the rotator cuff muscles depend on proper scapular rotation during arm motion. The scapula is one side of the attachment for the rotator cuff, and if the scapula can't rotate during arm abduction (when the arms go away from the center of the body), the rotator cuff muscles will have to pull against a fixed attachment.

For example, the supraspinatus, the muscle normally associated with a rotator cuff tear at its tendon, attaches to the top part of the scapula (the acromion); when it contracts, it can pull the arm up to the side. In response, the bottom point of the scapula should rotate out and up. If the scapular muscles prevent further rotation, all of the burden of raising the arm is borne by the supraspinatus and deltoid. At some point, the supraspinatus can't pull any farther without the humerus running into the acromion. This can overload the supraspinatus, causing trigger points and even damaging its tendon due to acromial impingement. A typical medical professional might diagnose this pain as a rotator cuff tear (even if no tissue damage exists), but it was caused by a muscular imbalance.

All of the stabilizing shoulder muscles must work together like an orchestra in concert for arm movements to have proper range without pain. This occurs because muscular imbalance in the highly mobile shoulder is dangerous, and the body responds by inhibiting movement, thus developing trigger points.

Our treatment planning must look beyond the prominent present- ing muscle at the outset and address the functional relationships in the region, with the aim of bringing balance to each functional muscle pair. In the shoulder, we begin our protocol with a focus on restoring scapular mobility due to its profound effects on the health of the rotator cuff muscles.

Satellite Referral in Practice:
IT Band Pain and Sciatica

Any gym is littered with people using a foam roller on the outsides of their thighs, where the iliotibial tract—often called the IT band—runs from the outside of the hip to the outer knee. This is simply another example of "rubbing where it hurts," which in this case is pain radiating down the leg, perhaps focused at the knee. Lateral leg pain usually invites misguided "diagnoses." This pattern may also be identified as a symptom of sciatica. Not uncommonly, the patient, perhaps with the input of a doctor or therapist, interprets their combination of poor adduction, tight hips, and a sciatic distribution down the lateral leg as a "tight IT band" that requires stretching and foam rolling.

If that weren't enough, the web is full of many examples of "the best IT band stretches," which are complete nonsense. This misinformed view that we can stretch our IT band is supported by nearly every personal trainer, running partner, massage therapist, yoga instructor, and movement professional and is very popular in the sports and workout worlds.

To discover the true source of the pain, we need to look at what's happening through the lens of trigger points and satellite referral.

You Can't Stretch Your IT Band, nor Do You Want To

A gross misunderstanding of anatomy is built into these assumptions. The IT band isn't a muscle but rather connective tissue. Physiotherapist and chiropractor Greg Lehman says the IT band "may be stretched in the short term due to its viscoelastic properties," but any "actual lengthening would require you to damage your IT band to get it into a lengthened state. Five minutes on a foam roller or ten minutes of daily stretching would not be able to do it."[27] Given that the iliotibial tract is an extremely tough body of connective tissue that provides the TFL and gluteus maximus a strong lever to move the leg and stabilize the knee, stretching the IT band itself would be a very bad idea, even if it were possible.

Some therapists very much believe in an "IT band syndrome" that involves lateral and local inflammation near the knee. It is popular to describe this condition as a "friction syndrome," but such an occurrence is not medically supportable. John Fairclough and his colleagues suggest in a paper from 2006 that the IT band "cannot create frictional forces by moving forwards and backwards over the epicondyle during flexion and extension of the knee" and that "ITB syndrome is related to impaired function of the hip musculature and that its resolution can

Fig. 6-3.
Ober's Test QR code.

27 Greg Lehman, "The Mechanical Case against Foam Rolling Your IT Band. It Can Not Lengthen and it is NOT Tight," *Reconciling Biomechanics with Pain Science*, March 17, 2012, http://www.greglehman.ca/blog/2012/03/17/stop-foam-rolling-your-it-band-it-can-not-lengthen-and-it-is-not-tight.

only be properly achieved when the biomechanics of hip muscle function are properly addressed."[28] Despite this study, most practitioners overlook the realities of the muscle. The hip abductor fibers of muscles like the gluteals and TFL are the anatomical elements most likely to limit adduction of the leg on stretch, along with painful referral down the leg.

The iliotibial tract has extensive fascial attachments to the femur along its length and is essentially just the lateral, thickened portion of the fascia lata, which is a fascial bag that envelops the thigh. The IT band itself does not and cannot limit adduction, which is often clinically evaluated via Ober's test, which is more accurately described as a test of piriformis and posterior gluteal fiber length. Ober's test assesses the ability of the femur to adduct and drop to the floor in side position. The abductor muscles of the hip are in a position to limit this test, and taut fibers due to trigger points in those muscles will keep the muscle short, cause referred pain in the glutes, hip, low back, and down the leg, and resist stretch unless the tender points are treated. Because muscles under stretch tend to refer pain if they have trigger points, when you do this stretch, you are likely to feel pain radiating down your leg over the area of your IT band. This, of course, reinforces the illusion that it's the IT band that you are stretching, but it isn't.

Where the Pain Originates

An experience of pain over the palpable IT band is misleading. Most people (including medical practitioners) tend to assume that pain is "in the local tissues." That said, those who continue to roll out the IT band in an attempt to stretch may find some temporary relief. However, the pain usually returns after a short time.

Rolling the lateral leg on a foam roller has little impact on the IT band itself, but for those who find rolling beneficial, they might be unknowingly treating myofascial trigger points in the vastus lateralis

28 John Fairclough, et al., "Is Iliotibial Band Syndrome Really a Friction Syndrome?" *Journal of Science and Medicine in Sport* 10, no. 2 (April 2007): 74–76, https:// doi.org/10.1016/j.jsams.2006.05.017.

(VL). If the VL itself has been a subject of acute overload, that would be an appropriate treatment if combined with range of motion work. VL trigger points can cause localized lateral knee pain that is very similar to the symptoms associated with IT band syndrome.

It is far more common for people to have chronic issues with the gluteal fibers and tensor fascia latae (TFL) because of their intimate involvement and sensitivity to gait disturbances. The gluteus minimus refers pain to the VL, so the pain will remain or return until the minimus is dealt with directly, no matter how much someone rolls out their lateral leg. In addition, the TFL might be referring pain, and the quadratus lumborum might also be involved if someone has a leg length difference.

In most cases, once again, satellite referral is likely hiding the true source.

Treating Lateral Leg Pain Patterns
Treating trigger points in the hip muscles is a much more sensible approach for lateral leg pain. It is often useful to initially compress tender points in the gluteus medius, gluteus minimus, and TFL with these muscles in a relatively shortened position. In people with these complaints, hips tend to get taut and hardened, making the muscles difficult to treat under stretch and also likely to contract on the short. Mechanical pressure during shortening followed by post-isometric relaxation is excellent therapy for these muscles. For a real-life example, see Doug Ringwald's case study in the blog section of coachingthebody.com on treating sciatica in a single session by addressing gluteal trigger points.

By treating the hip and VL muscles first, followed by progressive stretching, the client is likely to see a quick reduction in lateral leg pain and increased adduction, all without stretching or foam rolling the IT band. Rolling the hips with a lacrosse ball followed by adduction stretching is likely a far better use of the client's time than rolling the lateral leg.

Another factor to consider is leg length discrepancy, which often sets up one-sided leg pain. In these cases, the hips present at different heights when the patient is standing, causing the QL muscles to be at different lengths when resting. The QL on one side will tend to take on the dysfunction (usually on the side of the hip that is higher), and the QL might adaptively shorten to take the curve out of the spine as it ascends from a tilted sacrum. Part of the adaptive shortening includes the development of trigger points and taut fibers.

I include this example because these misdiagnoses and consequent experiences of long-term sciatic pain are very common. The solution, using the principles that I described, is quite straightforward, but it does require a significant change in world view on the part of practitioners. It saddens me to see so many individuals approaching us for help with their pain who have been let down by the system—which is one of my primary reasons for writing this book.

"As a director and filmmaker, I often find myself in unfamiliar places doing awkward things. I was filming in a moving vehicle in the front passenger seat when I turned left, and something in my left shoulder and neck area popped. It progressively worsened over a period of three years as nobody could fix it, and I was losing feeling in my left arm. Over the last six months, it started to become a throbbing pain in the evenings which would lead me to roll around the floor in pain, not knowing how else to cure this issue. A friend recommended that I call William Baird at the CTBI Clinic. I went in for a consultation and treatment. He explained to me that it was actually a muscular issue more than a nerve issue. We went through intensive deep tissue treatments for a few months, and incredibly, he fixed what could not be fixed! The pain in my left shoulder is gone. I am no longer losing feeling in my left arm. I can honestly say that this treatment changed my life! His understanding of how to listen to the issues, read the body's signs and treat the problem is at a level most people will never achieve. He is a special kind of person. I am lucky to know I have him there if I need him again!"

—Anonymous patient of Will Baird,
CTB advanced practitioner

CHAPTER 7

Coaching the Body Principles

Overview of CTB Principles

Coaching the Body is much more than a set of bodywork techniques. What makes this system so successful in relieving pain is a set of principles that we use to design our techniques and protocols. My years of working to apply the Thai massage techniques that I studied to the task of resolving pain showed me that understanding the true nature of pain and the role of the CNS is far more important than any particular technique or tool. Here is a summary of our most important guiding principles:

Protection: The CNS is preeminently concerned with protecting the integrity of the musculoskeletal system. In the presence of danger from heightened nociception, real or perceived injury, pain, imbalance, or joint instability, the CNS will take steps to protect the system from further threat.

Stabilization: The CNS uses muscles to stabilize joints as a protective response to perceived injury or excess mobility (splinting). Trigger points and taut fibers are a means of adding stability from muscles without an excessive increase in energy demand because of the nature of contractures, which are static and do not require constant input in the form of ATP. These compensations are hidden, "split off" from conscious control, and must be brought to light during therapy.

Nociception: Trigger points are a significant source of nociceptive input to the CNS, whether they are latent or active (producing direct pain referral). This nociceptive input can cause peripheral and central upregulation, heightening the sense of perceived danger and injury within the CNS and leading to a vicious cycle as the CNS attempts to stabilize and splint, creating more taut fibers, more nociception, and more pain. This can lead to regional pain syndromes involving reduced mobility and dysfunction in many muscles.

Regulation: Our primary goal in therapy is modulating the central and peripheral sensitivity of the CNS by treating networks of trigger points and providing the CNS with experiences of pain-free movement. This creates a beneficial cycle of downregulation, release, decreased pain, and improved mobility. We use neurological hacks such as distraction, vibration, EPS, and muscle energy techniques to provide dramatic shortcuts to downregulation.

Distraction: We minimize the tendency of the CNS to upregulate in the presence of discomfort and danger by providing consistent and broad distractive input during therapy in the form of touch feedback, therapeutic vibration, and stimulation from the EPS.

Movement: Joint movement and stabilization is a central function of muscles, and the CNS is highly sensitive to muscular disturbance and pain during movement. Treating muscles with movement and distraction is the fastest and most effective way to downregulate the CNS and release trigger points.

Networks: Muscles operate in hidden, extensive networks of functional relationships and satellite referral. Treating single muscles in isolation is rarely effective. Finding and treating the true origins of pain requires fully understanding these relationships that propagate chains of dysfunction and structuring the therapeutic approach to treat the significant related muscles in the correct order for a given pain pattern. The CTB protocols incorporate this knowledge.

Perpetuation: The muscular system doesn't simply malfunction without any reason. Underlying reasons may include systemic disease, injury, and, most commonly, simple anatomical and life-style variations that create chronic imbalance. Unless perpetuating factors are identified and corrected, dysfunction will return.

Now, let's explore why these are our guiding principles and how they work together to help us understand and interrupt the generation of pain at its true origins.

How Protection Can Go Wrong

The injury-centric attitude that pervades our medical system and many manual therapy approaches assumes that all pain is due to some level of injury. Hardened areas in muscle tissue (taut fibers) are conventionally thought of as "scar tissue" or "adhesions," and the job of the therapist becomes one of repairing injury and breaking up these hardened or adhered areas of fascia. Why these "injuries" happen and how simple manual therapy can remediate them is not well understood. As I have explained previously, this worldview also tends to emphasize focusing locally on the area of perceived pain, generally failing to achieve lasting pain relief.

Once we understand that the CNS generates the sensation of pain as an output based upon an internal assessment of danger (nociception), then it seems much more rational to address the parts of the system that are producing the nociceptive input and to downregulate the parts of the CNS that have become sensitized than it is to "rub where it hurts." Nociception can come from injury, but it can also come from trigger points, which are not injuries.

Over the course of my clinical work, I have come to appreciate the degree to which the CNS is constantly monitoring the state of danger in the system and using muscles to protect against further "injury." Non-disease–related chronic pain is no longer connected to the original insult (which may have simply been from trigger points and not an actual injury). Trigger points themselves can be a useful way to splint and stabilize joints.

By understanding the role of the CNS as protector, our therapeutic approach becomes a process of helping the CNS understand the true physical state of the body rather than fixing injuries (hence the name Coaching the Body). Releasing trigger points reduces the nociceptive load, while facilitated movement with distraction reeducates the CNS, causing it to lower its protective vigilance and hypersensitivity. We are essentially demonstrating to the CNS (and to the client's conscious awareness) that there isn't actually an injury, just a series of compensations that have resulted in trigger points, nociception, and pain.

Many situations can cause the CNS to develop a series of compensations that result in pain. Excess mobility and laxity in one or more joints, imbalances caused by anatomical differences or postural distortion, and temporary acute overload resulting in changes in function or posture are all examples of seemingly innocuous stimuli that foster a chain of events resulting in pain, possibly severe pain—and nowhere can an actual injury be found.

MOBILITY AND INSTABILITY

We tend to associate mobility with functionality. We might envy someone, perhaps a dancer or yogi, who is extremely flexible because they seem so much more fluid and capable than someone who is stiff and can't put their foot above their head.

Yet flexibility and mobility have limits. Highly mobile structures are, by definition, less stable. To use our tent analogy, a tent that isn't tightly stabilized by bungee cords can easily blow over in the wind. Some mobility is definitely beneficial, as with buildings built in fault zones that are designed with rollers so they move in an earthquake rather than split and shatter. The most stable structures have enough flexibility to avoid shattering under stress—too much flexibility, and they simply fall apart.

As a bodyworker who has worked with many dancers, yogis, and athletes, I came to understand that flexibility definitely doesn't equate to freedom from pain. In the human body, flexibility can come from two places: muscles and connective tissue. Ligaments and other connective tissue are designed to stabilize bony joints so muscles don't have to carry 100 percent of the load to keep the body intact. Ligaments are not significantly contractile and can only change length by 4 percent or less. Ligaments can't tighten themselves, and they don't stretch without injury.

Many individuals who become dancers and yogis innately have flexible joints because their ligaments are longer than the average person's.[29] This can bring with it more vulnerability to injury, so the body in these cases will tend to be more vigilant and protective. In this regard, flexibility does not equate to health. In the case of hyperpronation—a symptom of hypermobility in the bones of the ankle—muscles up and down the kinetic chain will overwork in an attempt to stabilize.

The primary tool that the CNS has to protect bones and joints from injury due to hypermobility is the muscular system. Muscles contract and shorten their length upon receiving signals from motor neurons, requiring energy to do so. Ligaments do not contract or shorten in this same way. So, while muscles can be effective stabilizers, they are not energy efficient. And muscles

---

29 I attended a workshop with yoga teacher John Friend many years ago, when he was early in his career. He made a statement that I found fascinating. He said that he could get a musclebound bodybuilder flexible more quickly than he could make a hypermobile person strong. And both strength and flexibility are necessary to safely traverse the challenges of yoga and life.

with less bulk and strength are more likely to become overloaded in the effort of attempting to stabilize joints with hypermobile ligaments.

MUSCLES AND PROTECTION

As I talked about in Chapter 4, the body creates taut fibers and trigger points that do not require continuous energy to stabilize joints. Dr. Leon Chaitow suggested the potential usefulness of taut fibers and trigger points in providing stability to joints:

> Simons et al. (1999) have shown that, in the absence of adequate levels of adenosine triphosphate (ATP), and in the presence of calcium, the actin and myosin elements of muscles are designed to lock in a shortened position. Trigger points therefore function effectively in the absence of ATP (thereby displaying an economy of resources), and as they are often strategically located in tissues that are straining to accommodate dysfunctional posture, or habits of use, they might be seen as part of the solution in some instances, rather than part of the problem.[30]

While the taut fibers have some downsides (primarily their tendency to trigger referred pain), their ability to provide energy-free stability to a joint that is perceived as injured or unstable has definite utility. The "energy molecule," ATP, is necessary to release the actin and myosin bonds, and in the absence of sufficient metabolic exchange, these fibers remain locked, forming a "virtual ligament" with low energy requirements. Sometimes this

---

30 Leon Chaitow, "Might Trigger Points Sometimes Be Useful?" Leon Chaitow, accessed September 18, 2020, https://leonchaitow.com/2009/04/14/might-trigger -points-sometimes-be-useful/.

process of the body using muscles to provide stability via chronic engagement is called splinting because it's as if the CNS is using muscles like a physical splint to stabilize a joint.

Evolutionarily, the pain generated by these taut fibers could be seen as a positive because pain is a way for the CNS to announce the presence of danger and discourage motion. In the case of an actual injury, mobility is dangerous in that it could exacerbate the injury. In an ideal scenario, muscular robustness and strength are a far better offset to hypermobility, but this requires first rehabilitating the overloaded fibers and then undertaking a careful, incremental program of building tone and strength without pushing the fibers into trigger points, pain, and failure.[31] In more severe cases, the body undertakes a more complete project of muscular splinting by embedding trigger points in functional units on both sides of a joint. This can result in severe immobility, a situation that then can be interpreted as "fascial adhesion" to a medical practitioner.

For example, frozen shoulder syndrome is a diagnosis that most people equate with adhesive capsulitis, meaning that fascial changes have occurred, gluing damaged tissues together so that range is practically eliminated. However, by using the CTB approach and viewing this condition as an adaptive protective strategy, we can reverse these symptoms in a relatively short time, which is evidence against it being a fascial adhesion.

Just because joint movement appears to have hard limits and excessive pain does not mean that fascial adhesion is the primary cause. If that were the case, we would have far less success than we routinely do at regaining pain-free range of motion in a session or two with patients who come in with the frozen shoulder diagnosis.

---

31 We include corrective exercise in our CTB protocols. By employing CTB concepts, individuals can train without generating excessive muscular overload and reverse temporary training-related trigger points with simple self-care techniques.

Fascial adhesions don't change in minutes of bodywork, but taut fibers are perfectly capable of letting go in that time.

To take a higher-level view of this perspective on the development of pain, it's a matter of seeing the CNS as an intelligent strategist, attempting to shore up the body's defenses against danger, as opposed to an opaque machine that just randomly breaks.

"SPLITTING OFF" IN THE BODY

Understanding the role of CNS as protector also dictates how we approach therapy. The coaching model consists of helping the body understand that the need for protection is mistaken, rather than overpowering damaged tissues and fixing what is "broken." We strive to understand the process that the body took to add layers of protection to a joint. These processes have become hidden but reveal themselves as we engage with the muscles, gently encourage movement, and listen to how the muscles react.

There are parallels to this process in trauma therapy. If a PTSD patient can re-experience the trauma in a safe, controlled way, the nervous system can begin to relax the protective holding patterns that it put into place to keep the trauma at bay and retain some measure of function. However, trauma victims may lose any memory of an event or compartmentalize it in a way that causes them to change their behavior toward others in an irrational way. This is known as "splitting" or "splitting off." Therapy must gently allow their psyche to re-experience the reality of what happened before true healing can take place.

There is a cost to the splitting off of a part of the psyche that occurs in these situations, but also a clear benefit. It allows the organism to carry on and be at least partly functional without constant crippling emotional pain. I see this emotional splitting off as analogous to what happens in the way the CNS manages the physical response to pain by locking down and splinting muscles.

One can see a protective logic at work here. Protection against injury occurs at the expense of reduced movement, fluidity, and, potentially, pain. If the psyche allowed the impact of a deeply traumatic psychological injury to be constantly present in the conscious mind, it would be crippling. Better to split it off and hide it away, even at the expense of a loss of fluidity and ease in daily life.

In the current biopsychosocial understanding of chronic pain, the brain monitors threats from the environment, nociception from the periphery, and emotional pain to make its overall assessment of "how dangerous is this, really?" All of these areas together contribute to the neuroplastic changes that can set up ongoing chronic pain as a response long after the original insults have faded out of memory.

The key to this insight is that instability and referred pain are perceived by the CNS as a threat in the same manner as psychological pain. If the organism were entirely self-aware, we might hope that because the pain response was, in a sense, self-generated, the system could just self-correct and ignore it after the acute phase and unwind the lockdown mechanism. But for better or worse, our human evolution has led us down a path of compartmentalization for the sake of preserving ongoing function.

Satellite referral reveals that, in some manner, the "output" experience of pain can cycle back and become an input. Referral that lands geographically over a muscle can cause that muscle to develop trigger points, which then generate nociception and a new pattern of referral. In essence, the body forgets where the original stimulus originated and reacts to the experience of pain as if it was due to local injury.

This tendency to self-protect and lose sight of the original stimulus is the central motivation for why we call this approach Coaching the Body. We provide inputs that make the body aware of the original source of the pain response, along with the compensations that have been put into place and stuck.

The Importance of Movement

Trigger point therapy, as initially described in Travell and Simons, focused on mechanical disruption of the trigger point area via injection as the primary treatment modality. This was then ideally followed by active range of motion work and/or spray and stretch. In actual practice, many therapists focused only on the disruption of the trigger points and failed to do the movement work. Clair Davies initially didn't see the value in stretching, and his original *Trigger Point Workbook* focused on the cross-fiber compression.[32]

In this interpretation, the trigger point is really the focus as "the pathology." If we get rid of the "bad guy," the pain will go away, not unlike performing surgery on an injury. Both are oversimplifications in terms of modern neuroscience. The CNS plays an enormous role in all aspects of myofascial pain: its development and manifestation, its perpetuation, and how successful we can be in our efforts to eliminate it.

Human bodies are massively complex movement systems. We take for granted the many coordinated pairings of muscles that must collaborate, or we would move in a jerky, spasmodic way and hurt ourselves. Muscles can only contract or pull, and that contraction gives them a unique capacity to move the structures

---

32 It should be noted that in Davies's book on the condition known as "frozen shoulder," Dr. Simons wrote a foreword in which he emphasized the need for active range of motion after the therapy as a means of integration.

connected to their bony attachments. When they do contract, they don't work in isolation, but rather they require collaborative partnerships with other muscles with similar function as well as their antagonists (muscles that have opposite function). In order to move a joint smoothly during muscular contraction, there must be a muscle pulling back on the other side to control motion, like a checkrein.

Smooth coordination of motion also requires constant monitoring by the CNS, employing the muscle's antagonists to provide a fluidly adjusted pull in the other direction. Without oversight by the CNS, our movements would be uncontrolled and dangerous to our well-being. The CNS relies upon movement-sensitive sensors embedded in muscles to determine the overall state of health in the system. Normal muscle behavior cannot be determined by how muscles behave at rest but, rather, how they behave in action.

For this reason, treating muscles in isolation or in a static state without movement is, by its very nature, incomplete and ignores the role of the CNS. Travel and Simons recognized the importance of movement to some degree, which is why they recommended having the patient do active movements after injection to allow the CNS time to integrate the change. However, with a treatment modality like injection or dry needling, muscles cannot be moved during treatment, or injury would result. This made it necessary for Travell and Simons to introduce joint movement as a separate step, which is less ideal than movement simultaneously with the actual treatment.

A muscle with trigger points will usually exhibit dysfunction as it changes length. Stretching tends to bring out the referral pattern of the muscle, while shortening can cause painful contraction. However, we cannot separate the behavior of one muscle during movement from the other elements of its functional unit. As we move a joint, our target muscle may be lengthening as its antagonist is shortening. If any discomfort results from the shortening muscle contracting autonomously, this will cause the brain to begin to restrict movement by engaging the stretching muscle. While it is tempting to interpret this behavior as an indication that we have to do more work on the stretching muscle, our ability to make change in that muscle will plateau because we aren't addressing the shortening antagonist.

Trigger points report to the CNS via nociception that something is wrong in the local milieu of the muscle. That report does not equate to pain or limitation; it is simply nociceptive information, which the brain then decides how to interpret. The CNS determines whether pain and immobilization are appropriate responses based on its level of sensitivity. The neuroplasticity of the CNS allows it to alter its sensitivity on the fly. If we attempt movement and the shortening muscle's trigger points generate a cascade of nociceptive input, the CNS will shut down the movement by engaging the very muscle we're trying to stretch.

This is why movement during treatment is so important. If we provide some form of distractive input to the shortening muscle, we hack the system so that the CNS doesn't get the same level of nociception, doesn't upregulate its sensitivity, and allows the target muscle to stretch. The experience of pain-free movement, in turn, exploits neuroplasticity in a positive way by causing the CNS to downregulate its sensitivity. You always have to remember that everything you do during treatment, along with the result, is being watched by a vigilant protector. A big part of our task is to influence the CNS so that it drops its vigilance, interrupting the downward spiral of pain, which begets splinting, which begets more pain and limitation.

Treating Functional Pairs Together

Certain muscle pairings in the body are more prone to experience coordinated dysfunction on opposite sides of a joint. If one muscle becomes troubled with trigger points, its antagonist partner seems to as well. In my experience, this seems to occur most dramatically in muscles whose action and function are most directly opposed and which play a role in repetitive actions such as gait. One implication of this setup is that agonist and antagonist muscles must be treated and considered as a unit when working with the CNS to reduce pain. If the brain decides that the current level of danger in the area of a joint warrants protection, it will ramp up engagement on both sides, like shoring up the tent poles with tighter cords.

Treating muscles in tandem with their functional antagonists is a major key to accelerating tissue change because it directly addresses the coordinating role of the nervous system. The CNS monitors signals from both the stretching and shortening sides during movement. Disturbance in either muscle will tend to block successful treatment of its opposite because the brain uses the two together for mutual protection.

In any joint movement, there is a stretching side and a shortening side. Most clients and therapists alike focus on stretch when muscles feel tight, and pain is experienced during movement. In my experience, many muscles with trigger points are unable to shorten gracefully, and this blocks stretch more effectively than any dysfunction in the stretching fibers themselves.

In Practice:
Treating the Adductor Magnus/TFL Functional Relationship

The adductor magnus and tensor fascia latae (TFL) have a unique relationship. Both of these muscles have hybrid actions: adductor magnus is a hip extensor and adductor, whereas TFL is a hip flexor and abductor. Most people don't make these explicit movements often unless they're a dancer or yoga practitioner. However, these muscles act as a unit during gait (walking) and are highly sensitive to gait disturbance.

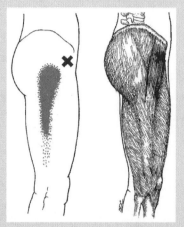

Fig. 7-1. TFL is both a hip flexor and an abductor of the leg, both of which oppose actions of adductor magnus. TFL trigger points may be misdiagnosed as bursitis of the greater trochanter.

From a biomechanical perspective, bipedal walking is a series of controlled falls in which the weight of the body continually transfers from one leg to the other. This results in one leg bearing the entire body weight as the other swings forward. During the weight-bearing phase, the body must maintain its balance while using hip extensors to push the trailing leg back and the hip flexors to bring the other forward. Additionally, the body must employ adductor and abductor actions to keep balance on the leg during weight bearing and prevent the pelvis from dropping as the other leg is off the ground.

Maintaining one-legged balance can be complicated by some anatomical variations that are quite common in the US population. If the ankle is hypermobile, there can be a tendency for the arch and ankle to fall in medially, a motion known as pronation. Some pronation of the ankle is necessary to walk smoothly. The term refers to a complex motion of the subtalar joint of the ankle when the ankle tilts medially and the front of the foot turns out.

If the subtalar joint has excess mobility, producing hyperpronation, the muscles of the foot, lower leg, and hips must engage to counter the tendency of the ankle to collapse and move weight to the outside edge of the foot. While this seems like a relatively minor effort, when repeated thousands of times per day, even powerful muscles like the adductor magnus and TFL can become chronically troubled. Other anatomical variations such as leg length discrepancies can add to the chronic load.

If they become overloaded, the TFL and adductor magnus can contribute dramatically to lower body pain, sometimes in indirect ways. The TFL refers pain laterally over the greater trochanter, extending toward the knee, resulting in a variety of misguided diagnoses, including trochanteric bursitis, IT band friction syndrome, sciatica, and the like. Adductor magnus can set up pain on the inside of the thigh through direct referral and produce medial knee pain via satellite referral.

To deal with lateral leg pain, patients are commonly told to roll their IT bands on a foam roller. However, they will find that even if they roll daily, the pain returns. This is because the issue is in the lateral hip in the TFL and glutes, not the place where they feel the pain.

Most therapists consider the TFL to be a difficult muscle to treat effectively. It tends to be a hard, gristly band. For a relatively small muscle, it has a big job to do in controlling the leg through the long lever of the IT band. What most people don't realize is that issues in the TFL are perpetuated in part by its silent functional antagonist, the adductor magnus. Unless you treat these two muscles together, you may find it difficult to get anywhere with either of them. The TFL also blocks full adductor magnus stretch via contraction on short; during treatment, you may encounter a hard end in the adductor magnus stretch and not know why or how to increase its range.

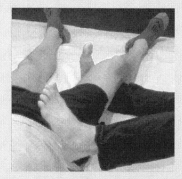

Fig. 7-2. Beginning TFL Treatment: Working into short.

It's very common for people to exhibit lateral leg referral and have no symptoms on the medial side of the leg. Even if a therapist is aware that the TFL and lateral glutes can produce a lateral sciatic pain pattern, they'll likely become frustrated when attempting to treat those muscles unless they understand the functional relationship with the adductors. This knowledge plays a role during evaluation, analysis of the issue, treatment, and follow-up. Without it, both therapist and client are doomed to repeating the same ineffective treatments every week, failing to create permanent change.

Our protocols incorporate our discoveries from twenty years of clinical practice and ensure that our students always treat functionally related muscles together. In this particular case, we first work TFL into short to assess and treat its behavior during shortening (which happens as adductor magnus is stretched). We then work adductor magnus into short and into stretch while also compressing the TFL.

Fig. 7-3. TFL Adductor Magnus Treatment QR code.

The Networks behind Chronic Pain

The great hope of trigger point therapy is that once we treat a point, the pain will vanish. Unfortunately, these situations are relatively rare. Sometimes a client might have a case of isolated, single-muscle referral, but these cases are primarily related to an acute event that happened to only stress one or two muscles.[33] More often than not, the muscle presenting pain is at the end of a

---

33 Falls and other sudden events can cause acute overload in muscles and quickly embed trigger points that cause significant pain referral. The referral can masquerade as injury-related pain, and its severity can feel very much like something was damaged. Even if there was damage, as the tissues involved heal, pain is likely to persist. At that point, the pain is from trigger points. If the acute overload was primarily in a single muscle and a therapist treats the trigger points and restores normal fiber length and tone to the affected muscle, the pain can be eliminated and never return.

chain of functional and satellite referral networks. If the therapist attempts to treat it as a single muscle activation, the results will be disappointing.

When we analyze pain in a client, we must work backwards from a presented pain pattern to what could be feeding it. As we just saw, trigger point pain is often the result of a web of interconnected muscles, which we call a network.

While this idea of interconnected networks of muscles may seem impossibly complex (and it was indeed very challenging for me to grasp when I was just starting out), the fact is that consistent patterns tend to recur across people and cases. You just have to be able to discover what muscles are most likely to be involved and put together a relevant treatment plan. To help you in this process, we've incorporated years of clinical observation into our CTB treatment protocols, making the treatment design process far easier for our students.

SATELLITE REFERRAL NETWORKS

In my initial studies of the *Trigger Point Manual*, I was intrigued by the mysterious phenomenon of satellite referral, in which a muscle becomes dysfunctional due to its position within the referral zone of another muscle. However, this idea wasn't as fully fleshed out as the other concepts in the books, and it was difficult to trace and connect referral patterns between muscles. Often the book would mention satellite referral in chapters that had little to do with the referring muscles. I had to do a lot of detective work to compile this information.

I began exploring satellite referral in more depth many years ago in my own practice. I found it to be much more common and pervasive than was conveyed in the original Travell and Simons materials. Over the years, I began to build our own catalogue of satellite referrals and continued to find that the phenomenon was a key factor in many areas of the body.

Satellite referral is not random, and it is highly repeatable. But because it can be entirely hidden or present at the end of a chain referral pattern, it is also mysterious and confusing. Just because it is hidden does not mean that it isn't there. Often, the beginning and middle of chain muscles along the source of the pattern have latent trigger points, so the client doesn't show any evidence of that particular muscle's pain pattern. Nevertheless, the pattern is still operating.

Example: Serratus Anterior

The referral pattern of serratus anterior goes over the shoulder blade and spine, directly over the low trapezius trigger point area. The low trapezius, in turn, can refer up into the high trapezius. Both trapezius and serratus anterior have a broad expanse and a wide range of fiber directions. Because the muscle sections have their own controlling nerves, the low, middle, and high sections of the trapezius and serratus anterior can act independently to move and stabilize the shoulder blade. In the case of the trapezius, trigger points in the low trapezius, which depresses the scapula, refer into the high trapezius.

This is a case of satellite referral within the same muscle. The low trapezius fibers must fight the tendency of the scapula to roll forward and protract, so the low and middle trapezius tend to be stressed if a rounded shoulder posture is present. This means many

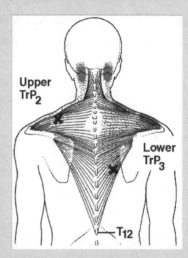

Fig. 7-4. The low trapezius trigger points refer into the same muscle but in the high fibers.

people tend to experience a constant flow of satellite referral from serratus anterior to low trapezius to high trapezius.

The high trapezius fibers have a very different function than the low fibers. They elevate the scapula. They are likely being subjected to satellite referral from the low trapezius, which further adds to the tendency of the high trapezius fibers to activate and shorten. This relationship is one reason why shoulder rubs feel good but don't have much lasting effect. The dysfunction in the high trapezius is being perpetuated by referral from the low fibers of the same muscle.

The situation gets more complex when we add serratus anterior to the equation. Not only does serratus anterior refer into the low trapezius, but I have found that the serratus is the muscle most responsible for protracted shoulder posture, rather than the pectoralis major. It tends to shorten and pull the scapula into protraction, which stresses the low/middle trapezius and rhomboid fibers, which are its antagonists. In other words, serratus refers into its functional antagonist (the low and middle trapezius), meaning that we have both a satellite referral and a functional relationship between these two muscles, which explains why we have found them to be so tightly coupled in therapeutic shoulder work. Even if the pain is felt in the trapezius, treating the trapezius without recognizing its connection to serratus anterior would not adequately treat any scapular positioning issues, and the functional distortion and satellite referral from the serratus will cause the pain to return, or perhaps never even fade.

The chain of muscles can be even longer. Serratus anterior can easily set up satellite referral through low trapezius to high trapezius and other cervical muscles. The high trapezius and splenii (in the back of the neck) alone can produce a vivid, crippling headache pattern. Because the configuration of protracted shoulder posture often accompanies a forward head and neck, which places excess mechanical strain on the posterior cervical muscles, this referral chain is quite common. It may seem far-fetched that a muscle on the side of the ribs could set up severe headaches, but I hope this explanation demonstrates how it actually is quite logical.

We at CTBI have documented clinically relevant satellite referral patterns throughout the body. Satellite referral is not a sideshow or some peculiar, unusual phenomenon. In my experience, it has direct relevance to the most common pain complaints that all therapists see. If the therapist isn't aware of how these patterns—often seemingly hidden—operate, they will fail to get to the source of the issue, and the pain will persist or return. That's why we incorporate our knowledge of satellite patterns into the design of our regional protocols.

Our protocols address the potential sources of satellite referral but also deal with the functional relationships. We need to be sure at each stage of treatment that we're dealing with all of the influences that keep each muscle in its dysfunctional pattern. Otherwise, temporary, incomplete results are inevitable. For example, if a patient pays us a visit for headache pain, it would be a mistake to just treat the direct referral muscles in the neck that cause headaches. In our upper body protocols, we always assess and treat scapular positioning disturbance. Serratus anterior and the trapezius are core muscles in any scapular positioning issue. Even just adding serratus to the treatment design of a headache session wouldn't be enough because it would fail to acknowledge the intimate functional connection of serratus anterior and the trapezius.

This discussion hopefully explains in some detail why I say that analysis and a firm grasp of the principles are far more important than technique. You can have all the fancy tricks and techniques in the world to get rid of trigger points in a given muscle, but if you apply them without considering the muscular relationships feeding the dysfunction, you will likely be unable to relieve your client of their pain in any kind of lasting way.

Where Functional and Satellite Referral Meet: Antagonist Referral

There are certain key muscle pairings in which referral and function overlap in a dramatic way. Returning to the serratus anterior and trapezius example, the referral pattern of the serratus anterior falls directly over low and mid trapezius trigger point areas. These fibers also happen to have an intimate functional relationship to the serratus, because they are its antagonist partners in moving and stabilizing the scapula. As we discussed, this can lead to a chain of referral terminating in head and neck pain, but their antagonist referral relationship also potentiates dysfunction in these paired muscles.

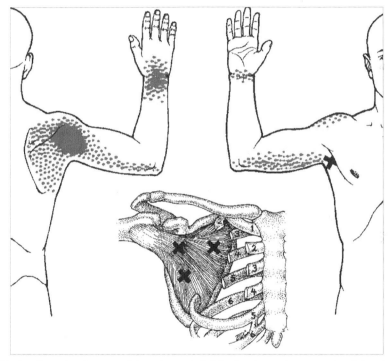

Fig. 7-5. The referral pattern of the subscapularis falls directly over its antagonists, infraspinatus and teres minor.

Serratus/trapezius dysfunction is seen in virtually every type of shoulder, forearm/hand, and head/neck pain. The serratus anterior tends to adaptively shorten and develop taut fibers, perpetuating rounded shoulder posture. As an antagonist to the serratus, the low/

mid trapezius is likely to become dysfunctional as well, becoming long and weak with taut fibers. As the serratus develops dysfunction, its referral over the trapezius will further compromise the trapezius. Thus, both sides enter a downward spiral of locked, protective engagement.

Another key muscle pairing that exhibits antagonist referral is subscapularis and infraspinatus. These important rotator cuff muscles are direct antagonists and are also both involved in stabilization of the head of the humerus in the shoulder joint. The referral zone of subscapularis is focal in the posterior shoulder, over the infraspinatus fibers. Not surprisingly, this pair usually shows dysfunction together. When neurologically-coordinated function and satellite referral coincide in antagonist referral, it creates a particularly potent combination that tends to accelerate the development of mutual dysfunction and keep it locked in place.

"Karen is an avid tennis player. She began having chronic pain between her scapula and spine and some sensation down her arm into her elbow. We began with CTB scapular positioning protocol, treating her pec minor with EPS and going through all the fiber pairings that were contributing to her scapular protraction. Within one session, she saw results! Karen is also someone who is on the go constantly. We began working with her breath because her ancillary breathing muscles, such as scalenes, were clearly stressed, and scalenes are a primary cause of interscapular pain. With coaching, she learned how to use her diaphragm to breathe instead of the muscles in her chest and neck. Within three sessions, she had 80 percent relief! She uses a lacrosse ball for self-care, and we do maintenance sessions once or twice a month. She has now added pickleball to her tennis regime. With CTB, she has increased ROM and decreased pain, and she can do what she loves."

—Nikelle Borough, LMT, CTB practitioner, and yoga instructor, Lake Geneva, Wisconsin

CHAPTER 8

CTB Protocols:
Intelligent Sequences

One of the most difficult tasks for a therapist is designing treatments based on the client's needs. Massage therapists learn fixed sequences, but sequences don't work when your treatment includes assessment and discovery of the true origins of the client's pain. In this chapter, I'll introduce the concept of CTB protocols, which I consider one of the most important contributions of this work. Protocols are guidelines with built-in decision points and branches based on what we find in the treatment.

For all of its depth as a reference, *The Trigger Point Manual* is not a useful guide for constructing manual therapy treatments. And, as I have mentioned before, I also found Thai massage sequences to be incomplete and their organizing logic sometimes opaque. Yet, as I received more invitations to teach bodywork, I realized my students needed useful rules for how to apply the many techniques and sequences I had been developing. In addition, many of my clients came to me seeking relief from pain.

I desperately wanted a set of protocols I could follow to help my clients. I wanted someone to tell me which muscles were most important, how they were connected through chains of satellite referral and function, and in what order to treat them. But that information didn't exist.

As a practitioner as well as a teacher, my chief dilemma was sorting out which techniques should be applied to a given pain condition and in what order. Massage therapists are usually taught to use sequences, but trigger point therapy has entirely different goals than typical massage therapy. Understandably, most of us began by doing the sequences as they were taught to us, making minor tweaks, and just seeing how it worked out.

But something important was missing: where pain originates. Sequences are less useful when you're trying to do detective work on which muscles are really contributing to the pain.

In the beginning, I would establish a set of muscles that could be causing the pain, and then I would attempt to determine a treatment order. Then I would try to use the techniques I had learned that seemed related to those muscles. It took years, but eventually, I was able to develop the CTB protocols as fully as they are today.

When I began integrating trigger point work into my Thai massage practice, a client would come in with a pain complaint, which I would have them draw on a body chart. I would then compile a list of muscles that were most likely to cause the complaint based on Travell's work, assigning some kind of priority to them because I might not get to all of them in a single treatment. Then I would have to decide on an order of events. I usually had the Travell books open in my treatment room, right next to my mat. It was nearly impossible to do all these things on the fly when a client had just come in, so I would ask them to send me the pain chart in advance.

Doing all of this analysis when a new client walks in and you're seeing their pain chart for the first time, remembering what muscles might be relevant from Travell and Simons, and then putting together and delivering a rational sequence of Thai techniques, all in the space of an hour or two, is virtually impossible for an inexperienced practitioner. My students and I (not to mention my clients) needed to work from a set of protocols, but they didn't exist. So I spent the next fifteen years of my life creating them.

My journey involved years of studying, seeing what worked, and discovering via hard experience how important the hidden networks of satellite referral and functional relationships actually were. And as my work began to focus increasingly on satellite referral and the critical functional relationships between muscles, the problem of treatment design only became more complex. I realized that it wasn't sufficient to just go down a priority list of muscles and treat them all and hope I had fixed the problem (which I often hadn't). I had to also consider the list of muscles that could be silently referring into each of the ones on my list, along with all of their functional antagonists. And come up with a reasonable treatment order that I could do in sixty or ninety minutes.

I divided the body up into seven pain areas based on the Travell and Simons divisions, creating treatment protocols for each one that followed a rational order for applying the techniques I had at my disposal to all of the muscles that might be relevant. The original versions of the seven protocols were somewhat complex because they included all of the possible muscles for each pain area. We had not yet begun to pare down the possible muscles to a set of the most common.

These were the seven pain areas:

- Head, neck, and facial pain

- Shoulder and upper arm pain

- Forearm and hand pain

- Mid back, thoracic, and abdominal pain

- Low back, gluteal, and pelvic pain

- Hip, thigh, knee, and groin pain

- Lower leg, ankle, and foot pain

We worked with these protocols for several years, and I began to realize that a much smaller set of muscles caused most of the reported problems in the upper and lower body. The "Pareto Principle" was very much in effect.

Simplifying Our Approach

The Pareto Principle, also known as the 80/20 Rule, named after economist Vilfredo Pareto, specifies that approximately 80 percent of effects come from 20 percent of the causes. When applied to a given situation, it can greatly simplify a system without sacrificing much in the way of accuracy.

When I examined the thousands of cases my students and I treated, it became clear that most pain comes from a limited set of muscles. There are outliers, but the vast majority of cases are very similar. Over time, it became clear to me that the 80/20 rule applied to my work. Even though patients show up with a lot of variation in their pain patterns, the underlying causes are usually similar. Apart from the acute cases—which are easier to analyze and also very much in the minority—chronic pain tends to originate from a small set of perpetuating factors that influence a common set of muscles. While the satellite referral chains can be several muscles long, the good news is that they are predictable and tend to recur across populations. This was good news for my beginning students, too, because I wanted to give them a smaller mountain to climb.

At the time, my clinical certification program required mastery of all of the protocols covering a list of 108 muscles in the body, many of them being smaller muscles in the head and neck, forearm and hand, and lower leg and foot. Problems in these muscles are less common than in the shoulder, back, and hip (mostly because of their function). For example, muscles in the forearm and hand control grip as well as wrist flexion and extension, and they are less likely to be causes of pain in the general population than the muscles in the shoulder. A carpenter or jeweler might put this set of muscles under greater strain than someone whose work doesn't require as much grip strength. However, the shoulder muscles often refer into the forearm and hand and are much more likely to become troubled in the average person.

Muscle by muscle, I carefully analyzed which ones regularly contributed to pain. As the 80/20 rule suggests, a small percentage of muscles are responsible for the vast majority of pain that we see in our practices. In fact, we found that there are only thirteen or fourteen key muscles for the upper body and the same number for the lower body.

In addition, I wanted to lower the barrier of entry for someone new to my program so they could learn the principles and relevant muscles and earn our basic certification level, Coaching the Body Practitioner (CTBP), quickly and be effective bodyworkers.

With that aim, I created two Core Protocols that would become the manual therapy focus for CTBP: Core Upper Body and Core Lower Body. Starting with this framework gives the therapist a high likelihood of success. The two Core Protocols are relatively easy to teach, and each covers the muscles in an order that makes sense for the vast majority of upper or lower body pain. They provide a sensible treatment order for the twelve to fourteen muscles that cause the most pain in the upper and lower body, based on our analysis of many client sessions. Following a protocol involves constant assessment and decision-making, tuning the protocol for each individual's needs.

We've now reorganized our system around these core protocols, and we cover the full body areas in our Advanced and Master certification levels. I'm now confident that our first-level CTBP students can complete that program in a year or less and be highly effective at resolving pain issues that baffle much more experienced therapists. Students of CTB don't have to work laboriously through all the possible muscles for a given pain condition or waste time on unimportant muscles; they also understand the contributions of satellite referral.

The protocols provide an optimal treatment order that takes satellite referral and functional relationships into account and can be completed in a single one- to two-hour session. They include the smallest set of muscles that contribute to the vast majority of pain cases. Protocols involve constant decision-making, eliminating unnecessary sections to maximize effectiveness and efficiency and allow more time to focus on the truly relevant muscle groups. The protocols and the method of analysis behind them are the most important knowledge in our teaching programs.

Protocols are organized into modules, which are related groupings of individual techniques for assessing or treating muscles and possibly their antagonists. A module is a discrete set of steps organized around a higher-level goal. Each module visits a specific muscle group, first focusing more on assessment than treatment. We apply treatment cycles to each individual muscle. For example, one of the most important modules in the Core Protocol for the Upper Body deals with normalization of scapular positioning: assessing scapular position and movement, then treating all of the functional pairs that move the scapula. Of course, there are always unusual and advanced cases for which the core muscles are not sufficient. We have a full set of Advanced Protocols that add a more complete set of relevant muscles to the basic framework of the Core Protocol. These seven full body area protocols deal with all of the less common muscles relevant to each pain area. They are, by necessity, longer protocols that require decision-making and triage to fit into a ninety-minute session, requiring more knowledge on the part of the practitioner. For example, the Full Shoulder Protocol follows the basic structure of the Core Protocol for the Upper Body but adds the other muscles relevant to shoulder and upper arm pain (twenty-six in all). The advanced muscles are relevant in far fewer cases but are sometimes needed for more esoteric cases.

Choosing the Appropriate Protocol

The first step in deciding how to approach a case and what protocol to use is the intake form.

We provide an extensive online intake form to our clients so that we can uncover all of the significant factors that might be contributing to the person's pain. The CTB pain chart is an online, interactive image that allows the patient to draw where they experience pain on their body. Accurate pain charts can be extremely important. For example, people don't just have wrist or hand pain; their pain might radiate from the arm, be ulnar, central, or radial, or only involve certain fingers. These details point to different muscles and should not be overlooked. We also ask about medical history, nutritional factors, a history and description of the pain, lifestyle factors, stress, exercise, work, sleep, and play.

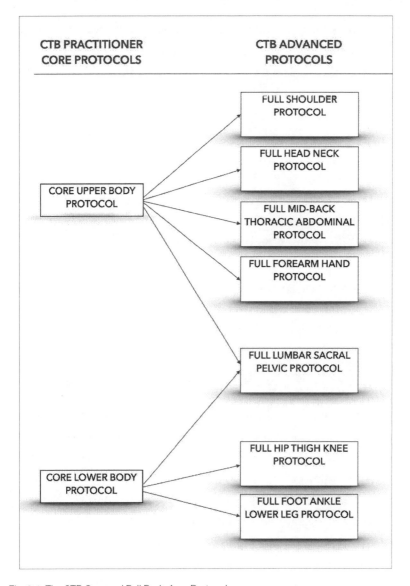

Fig. 8-1. The CTB Core and Full Body Area Protocols.

Body awareness varies greatly from person to person, and some patients may have a tough time mapping their pain accurately on a two-dimensional body image. If the patient draws circles or Xs on the chart, you will need to record a better drawing yourself when you interview them.

When you meet with the patient, ask them to describe their pain, how it came on, what it feels like, and what makes it worse or better. You should also observe how they sit, stand, and breathe. Do they tend to stand on one leg or cross one leg over the other? Do the muscles of their neck stand out as they breathe? These details can be extremely important.

The Core Upper and Core Lower protocols can each be performed in sixty to ninety minutes, including assessments. Efficiency depends on your experience and familiarity. Some clients may come in with clear upper or lower body pain. Some may have both, and they are usually related, but don't try to treat too much in a single session.

I generally pick one protocol if the client has pain in both. I sometimes start with the lower body unless their upper body complaints are very disturbing. Many upper body issues are sensitive to posture, which begins with the feet, so assessing the client for hyperpronation and leg length discrepancy (LLD) and doing a lower body treatment may well improve some of the upper body issues. A very skilled therapist can do a productive amount of work in both areas in a single session, but you need to have a good command of the material. In many cases, a smaller subset of the protocol can be done quickly and afford a lot of relief, in terms of both bodywork and self-care—but you have to understand what is most important.

The Core Protocols are the primary framework that we use to implement neuroplastic change and move the treatment strategy away from a sequence of individual muscle treatments toward integrated interaction with the CNS.

A Full-Body Pain Map

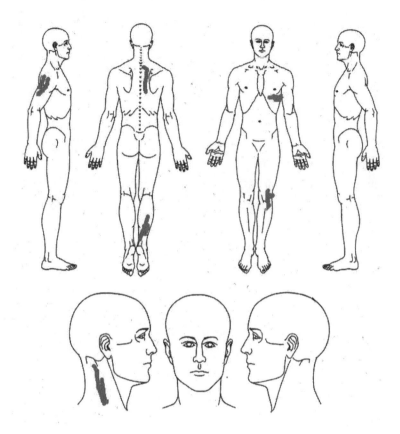

Fig. 8-2. Sample pain chart showing lateral asymmetry.

For example, the pain chart in the illustration shows a clearly one-sided pattern in the upper and lower body. My immediate suspicion would be a significant effective LLD. All of the symptoms in the leg and knee could be caused by a common satellite referral pattern that we see with LLD. Both lateral knee pain and posterior lower leg pain can be a result of gluteus minimus referring its lateral and posterior sciatica patterns down the leg. There might also be issues with the intrinsic muscles of the lower leg due to ankle and foot instability accompanying uncorrected hyperpronation.

LLD could contribute to upper body pain as well, via the scapular positioning muscles responding to LLD. In this case, I would look for protracted shoulder posture. Levator scapulae is very sensitive to shoulder elevation and would be a logical cause for the pain medial to the scapula. Serratus anterior is almost certainly involved, both in direct referral on the side of the chest and also referring into the low trapezius and then satellite referral to the high trapezius.

After you see these patterns in different forms in many people, you begin to develop a "radar" for what might be causing them. We form a hypothesis about the origins of the person's pain, which we must refine and modify as we gather each new datapoint about the person, their lifestyle, and how each muscle feels.

Based on this analysis, we could decide to do a lower or upper body session, depending on which pain complaint is most both-ersome to the client. In either case, we would assess and correct the lower body perpetuating factors (LLD and hyperpronation).

A Note on Analysis

I make a point of separating the analysis of the origins of a client's pain from the specific therapeutic approach being used. The analysis can be used in a variety of modalities. We've identified techniques and protocols for bodywork and self-care, making it possible for people to benefit from our approach with or without a therapist. We have had students successfully incorporate the CTB method into many different modalities, including massage, shiatsu, physical therapy, chiropractic, yoga instruction, Pilates, Gyrotonic, self-care, personal training, athletic training, occupational therapy, and more. We've even had great success working with clients remotely, helping them learn and apply appropriate self-care techniques.

Overview of the Core Lower Body Protocol

Treatment Modules: Lower Core	
1 Assess Assess Hip Rotation and Ankle Mobility	Supine
2 Crossover Stretch and Knee Assessments	Supine
3 TFL & Anterior Glutes Into Short	Supine
4 Tibialis Anterior and Soleus	Supine
5 Hip Over Knee—Glutes on Short; Assess Adductor Longus	Supine
6 Adductor Longus	Supine
7 Adductor Magnus	Supine
8 Quads & Hamstrings Short	Side
9 Hamstrings & Rectus	Side
10 Glutes Sitting Under and VL	Side
11 Extended Leg Position: TFL, Glutes, QL	Supine
12 Resolving Stretches	Supine

Fig. 8-3. Lower Core treatment modules.

The Core Lower Body Protocol begins by assessing the relative contribution of lower leg and hip muscles and goes into detailed treatment of adductors, glutes, quadratus lumborum, quads, hamstrings, and the primary movers of the ankle. The Core Lower Body Protocol includes fourteen individual muscles (see illustration), and some are more likely to cause pain than others. For example, the hamstrings and short quadriceps tend to be more influenced by satellite referral than having intrinsic dysfunction unless the individual is involved in activities that particularly stress those muscles.

Many lower leg complaints—including plantar fasciitis and various types of foot, calf, and ankle pain—derive from the same satellite referral patterns. In these cases, we must quickly assess the condition of the ankles because the tibialis anterior and soleus will often shorten to lock down the ankle and make it rigid in response to hyperpronation, while at the same time, satellite referral sends pain from the hip over the muscles of the lower leg and foot.

Based on the intake and interview, we hypothesize which muscles are the key pain contributors, using the protocols to constantly test, verify, and refine our hypothesis. We begin at the feet, which allows us to assess the condition of the ankles and lower leg muscles. Then we do some basic hip stretches that allow us to determine how the hips, adductors, and TFL might be contributing to the pain.

The rest of the modules focus treatment on the adductors, quads, hamstrings, and glutes (if indicated), finishing with some integrative stretches. All of the treatment modules work with agonist/antagonist pairs.

The Core Lower Body Protocol: Modules

The Core Lower Body Protocol includes twelve modules, and each module may consist of numerous techniques, summarized below.

1. ASSESS HIP ROTATION AND ANKLE MOBILITY

Foot, ankle, and hip mobility are critical indicators for what might be setting up lower body pain; both hypermobility and rigidity are problematic. This module aims to determine how much—if any—time we should spend on the lower leg and to what extent issues like hyperpronation and

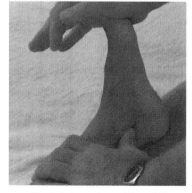

Fig. 8-4. Assessing ankle mobility.

LLD may affect the client's particular case. We assess hyperpronation separately with the client standing, and that can be done either before or after treatment.

2. CROSSOVER STRETCH AND KNEE ASSESSMENTS

The gluteus minimus is often implicated in pain patterns in the legs and is very sensitive to gait disturbance. For this reason, we need to understand its role in the client's pain pattern. Stretching the gluteus medius will generally cause the referral to become more intense, and the client is often surprised to find their radiating leg pain, knee pain, or even lower leg and foot pain reproduced by this stretch. The crossover stretch adducts the client's leg, which is the opposite action to the abduction role of the gluteals, so it's an excellent way to do this simple diagnostic.

Following the crossover stretch, we evaluate the condition of the knee and patella (kneecap). Knee pain can have local and remote components, so these assessments are meant to determine the relative importance of local muscles, such as the quadriceps. Vastus lateralis (the quadricep muscle on the outside of the thigh) can cause disturbed patellar tracking and chondromalacia patella (inflammation of the underside of the patella and erosion of the cartilage).

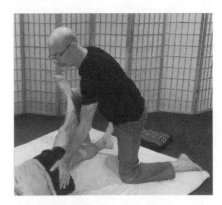

Fig. 8-5. The Crossover Stretch.

3. TREAT TFL AND ANTERIOR GLUTEAL FIBERS INTO SHORT

After assessing the gluteus minimus with stretch, we move on
to working the TFL into short.
The TFL is a very tough, dense
muscle that tends to become
chronically hardened by trigger
points and, like the gluteus minimus, is highly sensitive to gait
disturbance. Working it into
short with the heel or edge of

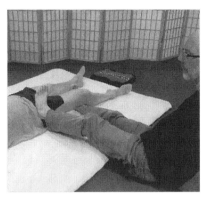

Fig. 8-6. Working TFL into short.

the foot can begin to soften these fibers so that later in the protocol,
we can stretch the adductor magnus without as much blocking from
the TFL, which may be contracting on the short.

As we abduct the leg, we put the adductor longus and magnus
on stretch, which may reveal some limitations in those muscles as
well. Following the work into short, another crossover stretch can
be used to provide some resolution for the TFL. For complete TFL
treatment, we can work more thoroughly in side position, which
provides for a lot more depth and control. This appears in the
Extended Leg module (#11).

4. TIBIALIS ANTERIOR AND SOLEUS TREATMENT

This section should only be done if you have identified lower leg
issues during the prior assessments. Hypermobility and hyperpronation can cause adaptive splinting across the ankle by tibialis
anterior, soleus, and other muscles that cross the ankle.

The setup for this module allows for both agonist and antagonist to be treated at the same time with movement through range
of motion, which is an ideal treatment scenario. Soleus gets firm
compression from the therapist's leg as you compress tibialis

anterior with the forearm.
Intersperse contract/relax
(more on this in Chapter 9)
frequently and loop back
through treatment to gain significant additional range of
motion. Tibialis anterior and
soleus can be worked into
short and stretch without
changing positions. For a

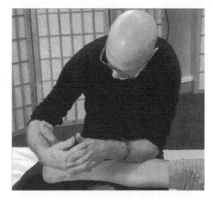

Fig. 8-7. Working tibialis anterior into short.

more complete soleus treatment, raised knee position can be used
with hooked fingers and a bent knee stretch. Ideally, this module
should be performed on both sides prior to evaluating hyperpronation, because it reveals the true mobility of the ankle. Ankle
rigidity is a common adaptation, particularly with older clients,
and can be responsible for poor balance and gait. It can be resolved
surprisingly quickly with these techniques.

5. HIP OVER KNEE: WORKING POSTERIOR GLUTES INTO SHORT

This is an important module that we always include in lower body
treatments. The setup with the glutes over the therapist's knee

allows working the glutes into
short in supine. We can also
immediately assess the degree
of protective engagement of
adductor longus, which can
be recruited as a way of pre-
venting painful contraction on
the short in the glutes. Based
on this sequence, we will have
a better idea of how much

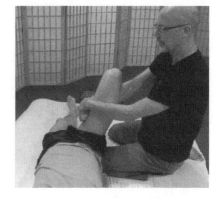

Fig. 8-8. Hip over knee.

time to spend on adductor longus in the next section. Adductor longus dysfunction can easily prevent the gluteal work from ever fully resolving glute activation. By leaning back, the therapist brings the leg into horizontal abduction, shortening the posterior glutes and piriformis and lengthening the adductors as it increases compression over the knee. Contract/relax should be used every few minutes, in both directions—leaning back to lengthen the adductors and pressing the knee across the centerline to stretch the glutes.

6. ADDUCTOR LONGUS

The adductor longus module is a critical part of the proto-col for many cases. The con-dition of the adductor longus will be revealed in Module 5, Hip Over Knee. If that module doesn't indicate that longus is engaging and/or contracting on short, this section can be minimal. If you find that the glutes cause shortening pain

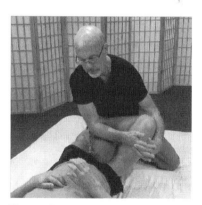

Fig. 8-9. A powerful technique providing broad compression from the shin during stretch or shortening.

when you try to stretch, you might first need to visit side position to work the glutes and TFL more thoroughly and do the adductor module after.

This is a typical example of how we create jumps and loops in the sequence of a protocol based on our findings during the session. The adductor/glute relationship is one of the most influential for lower body pain. We have numerous techniques in this module, all derived from traditional Thai poses, providing a wonderful variety of compression and stretch. We work in this module until the gains slow, and a plateau is reached, at which point gluteal work is indicated before further progress can be made. In the next module, we visit adductor magnus, which can throw referral into the adductor longus, a very common and important opportunity for satellite referral.

7. ADDUCTOR MAGNUS

Adductor magnus is very sensitive to gait disturbance from hyper-pronation and LLD and is a frequent hidden source of satellite referral into adductor longus. It functions in a close relationship with one of its primary antagonists, TFL. Both are often dysfunctional. We always work this large, dense muscle short first before attempting to stretch. TFL is likely to block stretch on shortening. Some of these techniques are designed so the therapist can provide feedback or vibration in the TFL while moving the magnus into more length. In severe cases, you might need to specifically treat TFL more fully in side position before being able to complete

magnus treatment. If you find the adductor longus to be re-sistant to treatment, adductor magnus satellite referral could be the culprit. Medial knee pain can be an indicator of this satellite relationship. It is quite common for magnus to refer into longus, which then refers into the medial quadriceps.

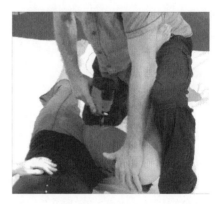

Fig. 8-10. Using vibration on adductor magnus into stretch.

8. MEDIAL AND ANTERIOR QUADS, HAMSTRINGS SHORT

This module represents a decision point. The short quadriceps are primarily responsible for thigh and knee pain; however, they aren't generally the most likely origin of that pain. Satellite referral from more proximal muscles is much more likely. We examine the person's lifestyle for evidence of strong quad use that could be directly affecting these muscles. In Step 1, we examined the knee and patella if knee pain was included in the client's intake. At this point, we would assess, based on that information and the nature of the client's pain, whether to even visit the short quads and hamstrings. We can work vastus medialis easily through range with vibration and the EPS in supine position.

Rectus femoris is a bit different because it also crosses the hip joint, and it can cause deep central knee pain. We work it into short and then in the Hurdler's Stretch under more length. Rectus femoris can also contribute to anterior pelvic tilt, so visiting this muscle along with TFL might be appropriate whenever there is pelvic tilt and an accentuated lumbar curve.

The hamstrings are similar to the short quads. While many people think they have hamstring issues, pain in the posterior leg is usually from satellite referral, which is why many therapists struggle with resolving hamstring issues. Functionally, they are also hip extensors and should be visited if rectus femoris is an issue.

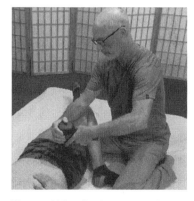

Fig. 8-11. Using vibration on rectus femoris in Hurdler's Stretch.

9. HAMSTRINGS AND RECTUS FEMORIS THROUGH RANGE: SIDE POSITION

We move into side position for much more in-depth work on the hamstrings and rectus femoris if those have been identified as important areas to attend to. We worked the medial side hamstrings into short in the last module in supine position. Side position is much better for the lateral biceps femoris hamstring group, so we begin by working those into short. We can then move above the

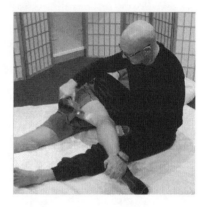

leg and work rectus femoris into short with 90 degrees of hip flexion, which will bring the hamstrings into stretch. Vibration is very useful on both sides.

This module is a detour that should only be taken if you have good evidence of actual dysfunction in the hamstrings or rectus femoris. Otherwise, skip this step and move into the glutes.

Fig. 8-12. Vibration on posterior hamstrings under stretch.

10. PRIMARY GLUTES AND VASTUS LATERALIS: SITTING UNDER THE LEG IN SIDE POSITION

Sitting under the leg in side position is our most important section in the lower core protocol. This is our primary treatment position for the gluteal muscles, which are implicated in most lower body pain conditions. We designed this treatment position to provide simultaneous feedback on the glutes and adductors, as it allows the therapist to change the length of the glute fibers via hip rotation. At 90 degrees of hip flexion, all of the gluteus medius and minimus fibers are medial rotators. If you raise the client's ankle, it brings the glutes into medial rotation, allowing compression into short by leaning into the forearm. External rotation provides a gluteal stretch in contract/relax.

This position also allows easy access to the vastus lateralis, positioned directly in front of the therapist's core. You can lean into forearm compression on taut fibers as you change length by opening and closing the knee.w Vibration is also an excellent choice.

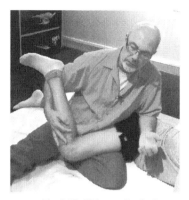

Fig. 8-13. Sitting under the leg.

11. ANTERIOR GLUTES, TFL, AND QUADRATUS LUMBORUM: EXTENDED LEG IN SIDE POSITION

The extended leg position switches the knees so that the top hip is in neutral hip flexion. This position makes the anterior glute and TFL fibers very accessible and allows for easy shortening and lengthening via abducting or adducting the leg. The therapeutic test known as Ober's Test is done in this position. As the leg is allowed to drop,

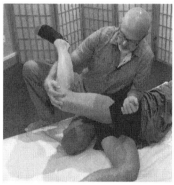

Fig. 8-14. TFL treatment in extended leg position.

it should be able to meet the floor or table without moving out of neutral hip flexion. This is a good test for TFL length because the TFL's role as a hip flexor will cause it to pull the leg forward as the knee drops to the floor if there are issues with range of movement (ROM) in that muscle. We work into short and length in these anterior fibers, which are well-known causes of lateral sciatic pattern referral.

The extended leg position is also the best position for treating the very important quadratus lumborum (QL). In side position, we can easily control the width of the pel-vis-rib space and, therefore, the length of the QL. We visit the glutes only briefly due to the fact that QL is so often a

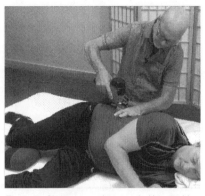

Fig. 8-15. QL treatment in extended leg position.

cause of satellite referral into the glutes and needs to be our primary focus. Frequently, the gluteal issues improve dramatically after we do some treatment on the QL. Vibration can provide a highly beneficial distraction in this sensitive area, hastening the release of taut fibers dramatically. Treating the QL is often able to improve all downstream symptoms in the leg, ankle, and foot.

12. RESOLVING STRETCHES

The muscles involved in lower body pain can influence a broad array of complaints, including low back pain, hip, and gluteal pain, and issues radiating down the leg, including the lower leg and foot. During gait, a lot of muscles must collaborate from the lumbar area to the ground. This extensive collaboration, combined with long satellite referral patterns, makes it necessary to reeducate the nervous system with some bigger stretches that involve many muscles. The Thai repertoire has some excellent techniques for this purpose, but we must choose them carefully for their effects.

One of my favorite general resolving stretches following the lower body protocol is the crossed-leg forward fold (covered in the next chapter). Crossed legs during hip flexion create a wonderful resolving stretch for gluteus medius and minimus, putting the legs into external rotation. The hip flexion will also provide some degree of gluteus maximus stretch, and the lumbar flexion lengthens the lumbar spinal erectors. We have many variations that can provide compressive feedback in the abdomen (if shortening problems are present) or that involve side flexion and/or spinal rotation. While many of the Thai stretches would have been inappropriate prior to the individual work on all of the lower core protocol muscles, at this point they can be very useful in allowing the CNS to significantly let go of its protective holding.

Overview of the Core Upper Body Protocol

Just as the QL, glutes, and adductors tend to form the core group that is responsible for most lower body pain, a key set of muscles commonly cause pain in the upper body as well. Some extremely common perpetuating factors cause these muscles to develop trigger points and become dysfunctional.

Hyperpronation in the feet and ankles often causes postural collapse, in which the torso and head move forward, putting additional strain on the posterior stabilization muscles like posterior neck muscles, iliocostalis, trapezius, and rhomboids. There is also a nearly universal tendency for the scapula to become chronically protracted and for the trapezius and rhomboids to become overpowered by the serratus anterior.

Compromised scapular positioning and motion can cause ripple effects throughout the upper back, neck, thoracic area, forearm, and hand. For this reason, scapular positioning protocol is at the center of our upper body analysis and treatments. As in the lower body, it's a mistake to place too much focus on where the pain is felt or to try and isolate the exact muscles causing direct referral. These muscles are at the end of a satellite referral chain and are involved in important functional relationships. This is why protocols are so important; they guide us through the foundational work that is not intuitively obvious when some of the muscular effects are hidden.

ID	Muscle Name	Primary Protocol
1	Trapezius—Upper	CU
2	Trapezius—Low/Middle	CU
3	SCM	CU
20	Scalenes	CU
21	Supraspinatus	CU
23	Infraspinatus	CU
24	Teres Minor	CU
26	Teres Major	CU
27	Subscapularis	CU
28	Rhomboids	CU
53	Pectoralis Major	CU
55	Pectoralis Minor	CU
59	Serratus Anterior	CU

Fig. 8-16. Upper Core Protocol muscles.

Most therapists who deal with shoulder pain have a tendency to overemphasize the muscles of the rotator cuff: the glenohumeral muscles that attach the arm to the scapula. These are end-of-chain muscles. Even though someone might be exhibiting classic referral from the subscapularis, jumping to that muscle to try to address the client's issues is invariably a diversion. The function of the shoulder muscles is much more important than their *action*. For example, the muscles of the rotator cuff share a common function, which is to work in concert to keep the humerus stabilized and centered in the glenoid fossa (shoulder socket) during arm movement. Each pair of muscles with opposing action must work together smoothly as the arm and scapula move. If the motion of the scapula is disturbed, all of the glenohumeral muscles and their antagonists are being given faulty information during arm movement. This can quickly progress into a regional overstabilization of the highly mobile shoulder joint, which many doctors identify as "frozen shoulder."

The Core Upper Body Protocol: Modules

Here is a brief summary of the five modules of the Upper Core Protocol. We begin in supine by assessing the rotation of the arm and observing any limitation from subscapularis and pectoralis major. Here, we can do some initial work on those muscles, but for full range of motion, we need to have the client in side position. Module 2 remains in supine, and we do initial work on the neck muscles. The muscles of the neck and cervical spine can strongly influence the shoulder muscles via neurological entrapments and/ or satellite referral.

We move into side position for Modules 3 and 4 because side allows for completely free movement of the scapula and glenohumeral joint. Module 3 is the centerpiece of the upper body protocol. We assess and correct the positioning and movement of the scapula, which, if protracted or immobile, can wreak havoc on the entire region. This is a powerful and unique sequence that, over the years, has revealed itself to be the key to correcting serious and long-standing shoulder, neck, and arm pain. This module came into being after we had developed and begun using the Muscle Liberator consistently. The speed with which the vibration was able to release difficult muscles like the serratus anterior made it feasible to develop a thorough progression through the fiber pairings of the scapular muscles and restore significant function in twenty minutes or so. The key to this acceleration is the incredible degree of neurological distraction provided by the tools.

Treatment Modules: Upper Core	
1	Assess External Rotation and Muscles of the Axilla
2	Assess and Treat Muscles of the Neck
3	Assess and Treat Scapular Positioning
4	Treat Core Glenohumeral Muscles
5	Return to Supine and Final Integration

Fig. 8-17. Upper Core Protocol treatment modules.

We do the movers of the arm last, including the rotator cuff. These muscles are far easier to treat once the CNS allows the scapula to move freely. Many therapists who know a little bit about trigger point therapy will jump to the direct referrals of muscles like infraspinatus or subscapularis and try to address them as the first order of business. However, they all cross the glenohumeral joint from the scapula, and when it doesn't move correctly, they are bound to be compromised—which is why we place so much emphasis upon the scapular positioning module. The protocol includes paying a brief initial visit to subscapularis, to assess and soften it. If intense referral from infraspinatus is limiting movement, we may choose to visit it briefly as well.

Finally, we return to supine for finishing work on the subscapularis and revisiting the assessments to determine what progress has been made.

1. ASSESS EXTERNAL ROTATION AND MUSCLES OF THE AXILLA

As the client lays on their back, we begin to assess their breathing and basic arm motion. With the arm abducted to 90 degrees and bent at the elbow, we move the arm slowly into external rotation to assess both range and quality of motion. If there are small stops and starts in the motion, that is a strong indicator of issues in subscapularis and infraspina-

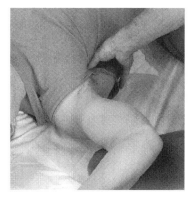

Fig. 8-18. Treating subscapularis and infraspinatus together in supine position.

tus. We also assess the degree to which any of the pectoralis major branches might be limiting arm movement.

This is a good position to do an initial assessment and brief treatment on the subscapularis and teres major, working into short and using movement with compression and vibration. We will return to more thorough treatment of those muscles after the scapular positioning module. Initial treatment on infraspinatus can be performed during Module 1 by placing the thumb in the subscapularis while the fingers reach around to the back of the scapula to treat infraspinatus with the fingertips during movement.

2. ASSESS AND TREAT MUSCLES OF THE NECK

From above the head with the patient supine, we can assess the height of each acromion above the mat or table. If we notice that the acromion is higher than normal or pulled in toward the neck, we will know to prioritize work on the pectoralis minor and clavicular pectoralis major as well as serratus anterior.

In the neck module, we treat high trapezius, sternocleidomastoids, levator scapulae, and scalenes, as well as the posterior neck muscles as a group. This work can help identify muscular issues that may contribute to forward head positioning, modified cervical curve, and excess engagement in neck muscles that could lead to compression and nerve entrapment. The neck is a potent perpetrator of trigger points and pain in the shoulder area and down the arm.

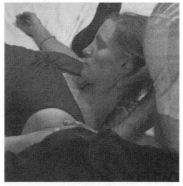

Fig. 8-19. Side flexion stretch for the scalenes.

3. ASSESS AND TREAT SCAPULAR POSITIONING

The scapular positioning module is the most important in the upper body. We identify fiber pairings in the large muscles that surround and move the scapula and normalize their behavior so the scapula can rest in a proper position on the back and contribute its share of rotation during arm movement. Muscles such as trapezius, serratus anterior, pectoralis minor, rhomboids, and levator scapulae, in addition to their critical functional role, have potent pain patterns of their own and are involved in satellite referral in the region. Muscles like infraspinatus, subscapularis, supraspinatus, and teres major tie into the scapula and easily develop dysfunction if their motion is disturbed.

The functional relationship between the low and mid trapezius/rhomboid fibers, which are scapular adductors, and the pectoralis minor and serratus anterior, which are protractors and abductors of the scapula, is the center of this section. Vibration is extremely important in this area due to the degree of neurological holding involved.

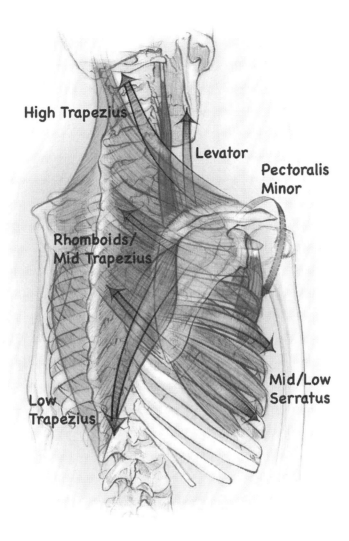

Fig. 8-20. Functional relationships between scapular positioning muscles.

If the patient has severely limited arm movement, this will make it difficult to adequately treat the serratus anterior and contract/relax many of the shoulder muscles. In this case, we visit the scapular positioning module and do what is possible before moving on to the glenohumeral muscles and then return for more scapular work. The scapular positioning module will restore some amount of scapular rotation, which will facilitate arm movement. The scapular muscles also can refer pain into glenohumeral muscles such as infraspinatus and supraspinatus, making it important to visit them prior to the muscles of the rotator cuff.

4. TREAT CORE GLENOHUMERAL MUSCLES

With improved scapular rotation, we can now move into treating infraspinatus, supraspinatus, teres minor, teres major, and subscapularis. We also observe scapular behavior and continue to integrate scapular and arm motion. Each time the CNS witnesses increased pain-free range of motion, this will help to downregulate the CNS

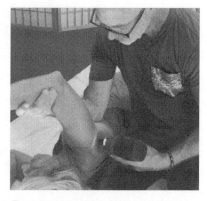

Fig. 8-21. Using vibration on infraspinatus and other glenohumeral muscles.

and allow for greater release. It's a way of demonstrating to the brain that no injury exists to protect or splint.

We begin with infraspinatus, holding the bent arm over our lunging leg so we can easily control the amount of external rotation. This allows working into short and eventually into a stretch position with the hand behind the back. If abduction is badly limited, we might need to tackle some work with supraspinatus and teres major first; they can be done in either order. Infraspinatus plays a key role as a humeral stabilizer along with the other muscles in the rotator cuff, and it is likely to develop ancillary dysfunction in any situation where the CNS has begun restricting shoulder motion due to perceived injury.

As motion improves, we use more integrative techniques, in which we try to provide feedback on as many of the shoulder muscles as possible while moving the arm. This is an important reeducation phase in which we can see positive neuroplasticity take effect and ROM increase dramatically.

5. RETURN TO SUPINE AND FINAL INTEGRATION

After thoroughly treating the other glenohumeral muscles, we return to supine to do final resolving work on subscapularis. This muscle is highly influenced by proper scapular rotation and the referral pattern of serratus anterior, as well as its strong functional relationship with infraspinatus. Subscapularis

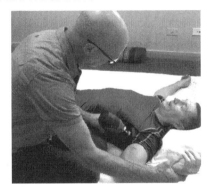

Fig. 8-22. Vibration on subscapularis after final return to supine.

and infraspinatus have an antagonist referral relationship—the subscapularis referral pattern falls directly over infraspinatus.

Supine is the best position for subscapularis treatment, and as in Module 1, we can also provide compression on infraspinatus by wrapping the fingers or thumbs behind the scapula. Generally, external rotation can improve dramatically at this step because of the greatly reduced influences on subscapularis and improved scapular rotation. In this step, it's common to see significant change, and patients are often amazed at how much their overall pain-free ROM jumps at this stage. We finish by moving the arm through various motions with as much feedback on relevant muscles as possible. The client then can begin to use active ROM and see how things have improved.

Summary

The CTB Core Protocols ensure that all relevant satellite referral patterns are uncovered to efficiently take out entire networks of trigger points, focus on agonist/antagonist functional relationships, and gradually build experiences of pain-free movement joint by joint, incrementally covering more movements and greater range. The protocols alternate between individual muscle treatment, invoking neuroplasticity via contract/relax, and gradually integrating movement with broader resolving movement.

We have been refining the CTB Core Protocols for many years, and they successfully address the vast majority of pain complaints that we tend to see in practice. The Core Protocols cover 28 of the 108 muscles in our muscle library. We cover the remainder in the Advanced Protocols, which build upon these Core Protocols.

In the first layer of study in our certification program—the CTB Practitioner (CTBP) certification—we train students to develop full competency in these core protocols, which generally takes students about a year to complete with both in-person and online components. Please see Chapter 15 (Resources for Further Study) for more information on how to learn the CTB Core and Advanced Protocols.

"Twelve years ago, I began my career as a bodyworker. I'll always remember learning in massage school about the average career span for massage therapists being five years. Five years? For the first five years as a massage therapist, I was definitely on that track of burnout! I would give the 'deepest' pressure massages. However, it wasn't really 'deep' work at all. I was delivering firm and intense pressure, yet I was missing the mark on two major aspects of productive bodywork: taking care of myself and taking care of the client.

"The first concept was so foreign to me that I was surely on my way to burnout! My self-care journey began when I decided to attend my first Coaching the Body weekend. I was so excited. I met so many diverse and interesting people. Every student was so eager to learn how to better serve others. It all starts with ourselves. I learned about metta, or loving kindness. Before I could truly help others heal...I needed to start the healing process. Finding forgiveness, compassion, and the utmost respect for what I do and who I am. Most important was the ability to treat myself with loving kindness or non-violence. The way I had been working wasn't serving my clients or me. Yes, they were receiving deep pressure, but they weren't releasing and retraining the body/mind to move freely without dysfunction and pain. Instead, I was attempting to assist the client in healing, but I was ultimately harming myself in the process. I did not understand the 'why' of the bodywork I was giving or that by working at the true source of pain, I work with more ease—and much more effectiveness.

"CTB was the lever of transformation in my practice—allowing me to bring awareness to self-love. Ultimately allowing better care for other beings! I began to learn different ways of holding my posture in the treatments. I was able to allow the tension in my body to let go and have more relaxed energy to give to my clients. I started using breathing techniques and meditating. Yoga became a regular practice in my life. I started practicing mindfulness. I began to practice and teach ways of deeply relaxing the body and tuning into the breath. By using these techniques, the parasympathetic nervous system can kick in, and releases begin to happen. And real change starts to occur. Brain maps are rewired. CTB is bodywork that really makes change."

—Nikelle Borough, LMT, CTB practitioner,
Lake Geneva, Wisconsin

CHAPTER 9

The CTB Treatment Cycle

The CTB treatment cycle structures our work with each individual muscle that we treat. In general, we'll follow the following procedure, understanding that we tailor the process to the specific characteristics of each muscle:

- Evaluate for taut fibers

- Initial softening with compression and vibration if necessary

- Work muscle into short

- Treat statically with electronic point stimulator (EPS) vibration

- Work through range

- Contract/relax

- Repeat until improvements begin to plateau

In this chapter, I'll outline the CTB treatment cycle. For more information, scan the QR code at the end of this chapter to see a video demonstration of the steps in action.

Evaluate for Taut Fibers and Tenderness

Palpation is the first step in identifying taut fibers, helping us determine whether to complete the remainder of the cycle or move on. Palpating for taut fibers must be done with knowledge of the muscle's fiber direction, strumming across the fibers at a 90-degree angle. Firm pressure is required to detect differences between fibers and to elicit twitch responses, both of which indicate trigger points. Tenderness may not be evident in the beginning because the tissues are superficially hard and desensitized. Because tenderness might be difficult to elicit in the beginning, hard, ropy fibers are the most reliable indicator of dysfunction at the outset, rather than tenderness. Vibration or cross-fiber strokes can help to soften the fibers. Tenderness often increases after one treatment cycle.

When fibers begin to soften and feel less tender, I advise students to strongly consider moving on to the next step. At this point, it's more efficient to move to other muscles that could be in a perpetuating relationship rather than banging away at a muscle that's showing diminishing returns. When I work with apprentices, I probably give this advice the most often: strive for progress, not perfection, and when progress slows, it's time to move along. Doing so, even if it feels difficult, will make the sessions much more efficient overall. Often, when you return to the muscle after visiting some closely related ones, it will have improved dramatically because you've addressed functional and satellite referral issues that are likely feeding perpetuating issues into the muscle.

In addition to palpation, we also use movement in our initial assessment. Moving joints is the most effective way to see how muscles behave in a dynamic environment of collaboration with other muscles. While it's gratifying to feel a taut fiber soften, softness alone isn't a sufficient criterion to assess healthy muscle behavior. Movement reveals any resistance to lengthening or shortening, as well as any pain responses that may occur at specific points in the arc of movement.

For example, at the beginning of our scapular positioning protocol, we move the scapula in a slow, circular manner to assess whether the scapular stabilizer muscles can shorten and lengthen in a smooth, coordinated manner. If the middle trapezius or serratus anterior fibers contract on shortening, it will cause a perceptible jump, in which the scapula appears to move on its own, revealing the dysfunction that keeps the scapula improperly positioned while perpetuating pain. This process is far more valuable than looking for active referral or simply palpating the relevant muscles for trigger points.

The presence of trigger points does not in itself determine whether the muscle will behave in a dysfunctional manner. Many muscles contain trigger points yet function normally. Some latent trigger points cause no perceptible pain but are quite potent at disturbing posture and function. For these reasons, we rely much more upon movement-based assessments than we do palpation.

Treat Statically with EPS/Vibration

Often following initial palpation, we need to soften the muscle. The muscle might start out with a hard protective shell, making it difficult to palpate even individual taut fibers. To help soften the muscles, we will use vibration, EPS, or both. With either approach, we treat a few points and then do contract/relax, and repeat the cycle. This is far more effective than trying to eliminate trigger points with compression alone.

When practicing Thai massage, I observed that the poses provided a great deal of stimulation to the CNS through several points of contact, movement, rocking, or shaking in addition to compressive techniques. All of these techniques effectively distract the nervous system. In an effort to adapt the distractive aspects of Thai bodywork to trigger point therapy, my team and I developed and began working with the Muscle Liberator, a powerful therapeutic vibration tool, which is essential for re-training the CNS.[34]

We have found over the years that certain muscles—typically the larger muscles—benefit from a period of overall softening with vibration, such as the gluteals, vastus lateralis, trapezius, spinal erectors, and adductors. Many people misunderstand the use of vibration and percussion tools in bodywork. They keep the muscles static and run the tool all over them, like a meat tenderizer. While this temporarily softens hard muscles, the lack of change in fiber length and failure to treat the muscle with its antagonists will make the gains fleeting.

More delicate, superficial muscles in sensitive areas—such as levator scapulae, scalenes, pectoralis minor, abdominals, and the more delicate areas of the forearm and hand—are best treated with EPS. Muscles that we address primarily with EPS are treated in a relatively static position because it's harder to move while

---

34 Sometimes massage therapists who don't know my work see our Muscle Liberator vibration tool and tell me, "You can't replace the hands or physical touch." They assume that we are trying to use a tool to do massage rather than the hands, which is not the case. The purpose of it is not to mechanically hammer out the tissues, and if it is used in this way, it will not be as effective and could cause bruising and other issues. Touch is critical in our system, but the hands simply cannot provide the level of neurological distraction of a vibration tool. And attempting to "rub trigger points out" with the hands, forearms, etc., is very hard work that lacks the critical distraction component.

holding the point (although with some muscles, it's both possible and desirable).

Working the Muscle into Short

Working into short consists of setting up our body position so that as we move the client's joint to shorten the muscle's fibers, we can apply increasing pressure with our body weight, rather than using excessive strength. Certain muscles tend to contract on short, which limits our ability to bring their antagonists into stretch. These muscles are typically good candidates for working into short, and for some—like the TFL, mid trapezius, and tibialis anterior—it's essential.

This phase of the treatment cycle varies a bit for each muscle, and we don't work all muscles into short. Some can't shorten completely due to the architecture of the relevant joint (such as the short quadriceps in the thigh, since you can only bend your knee backward, not forward), making it less likely that shortening contraction would occur.

It's important to note that the technique involves movement into short rather than shortening the muscle and then compressing it. We want to train the CNS as we're moving into the barrier where contraction on the short begins to happen. Firm compression or vibration as we move the muscle short can begin to change the CNS, whereas once the muscle has already contracted, the negative event has already occurred, and retraining is far less effective.

In Practice: Mid-Trapezius

Let's take a look at how, as a therapist, you would work the mid-trapezius into short. After assessing its behavior by moving the scapula, you work the muscle into short using a Thai/shiatsu technique known as cleaning the wing, done as follows. If the mid-trapezius area shows a tendency to contract on short, position your fingers like a blade with the scapula in a protracted posi-

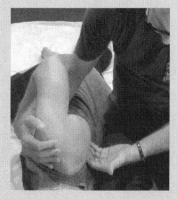

Fig. 9-1. Cleaning the wing—treating scapular adductors into short.

tion. Alternately, you can use your thumb if you can hold it rigidly stabilized. Then position the scapula with enough fiber length so that it has not yet contracted and remains soft. Hold your fingers rigidly like a blade, stabilized on your leg so your body weight does the work of moving the scapula.

Your fingers essentially provide an immovable object that the fibers of normal rhomboids would wrap around, allowing the medial border of the scapula to move over the fingers. At whatever point the rhomboid and/or middle trapezius fibers contract, they will harden and stop the process. You can adduct the scapula very carefully by leaning back and pulling the scapula toward the spine, but only so far as you can without the shortening rhomboid and trapezius fibers suddenly engaging. This requires careful attention and slow movement to firmly compress the fibers just at the point that they begin to contract. The increasing compressive feedback from the fingertips or thumb can defeat the tendency to contract, but only to a point. Each additional centimeter of shortening without contraction provides the CNS with an experience of more functional movement, allowing it to drop some of its protective guarding.

Work through Range with Compression/Vibration

Once the muscle has released enough to allow for some change of length, vibration with movement is highly desirable. The intense distraction provided by the Muscle Liberator can override the pain response that would normally cause the CNS to limit motion, helping us retrain the system out of the protective splinting it had fallen into.

Another version of this approach that we use in certain muscles, such as the glutes and quads, is to hold a compression point with pressure as we move the muscle through its range. In the glutes and TFL, we generally alternate vibration and compression. It's far easier for the therapist to hold a point and change muscle length than it is to keep the muscle static and move the compression. There may be one or two primary points of compression over specific trigger point areas in muscles we have identified as primary limiters of movement. In some cases, however, we may apply more general compression (which we call feedback) over several other muscles since so many must coordinate in areas like the shoulder.

It's important when moving a joint to have enough functional anatomy at your disposal to know which muscles are lengthening, shortening, and stabilizing and what their typical referral patterns are. Many massage therapists leave school and quickly forget their anatomy knowledge because they don't use much movement in their work. CTB therapists, to be consistently effective, must understand functional anatomy and fiber direction in each muscle because we rely upon being able to change muscle length. Unfortunately, this is not adequately conveyed in many teaching programs.

Feedback in the form of compression or vibration can be usefully applied in the trigger point area or in its pain referral zone during movement. In the referral zone, the feedback sensation will tend to mask and override the experience of pain. Without pain, the nervous system will more easily disengage muscles that were employed to splint and restrict movement. Our eventual goal is movement to full stretch without undue discomfort. At that point, the restricted sarcomeres will have pulled apart from their stuck contracture state and the muscle will no longer produce pain during movement, unless we failed to adequately address the antagonist.

Severe shoulder pain tends to be the most dramatic example of the effectiveness of incorporating movement with feedback during treatment. Patients may wince at even the suggestion of certain movements, so their CNS has become conditioned with burned-in pain pathways. We sometimes have to employ tricky positions, applying feedback with hands, thumbs, fingers, and arms to turn off as many muscles as we possibly can. This can be tricky, but there is a huge payoff. Long-standing conditions such as frozen shoulder can yield significantly in a single session when we adopt a stance of *coaching* the body as opposed to *fixing* the body.

Contract/Relax

Contract/relax is one of a class of "Muscle Energy Techniques" (MET) that developed in early osteopathic medicine as a means of influencing the CNS to allow taut fibers to relax and stretch more easily.[35] Tendons attach muscle to bone, and within tendons, golgi tendon organs (GTO) report the degree of tension on the tendon to the CNS. If you contract a muscle for several seconds, the pull on its tendon will increase, and the GTO will report this phenomenon to the spinal cord. But then, something very interesting happens: a temporary relaxation response occurs, which greatly aids in relieving the contractures of taut fibers containing trigger points.

I teach my students to intersperse contract/relax through the treatment cycle every few minutes. Compression and other treatment

---

35 Leon Chaitow, *Muscle Energy Techniques (Advanced Soft Tissue Techniques)* (London: Pearson Professional Limited, 1996).

modalities should be thought of as only the beginning phase of re-solving trigger points in a muscle. Contract/relax is a neurological hack that can create dramatic advances in a few seconds by facili-tating significantly more useful length in the muscle. The technique can be used on its own, but optimal benefit occurs when we use it following short periods of treatment with compression, vibration, or EPS. The stretch phase of contract/relax reeducates the protective CNS by providing increasing experiences of pain-free movement, advancing the stretch barrier each time it is done. It's a way of consolidating gains. After each contract/relax, you will find that the muscle is softer, less tender, and has significantly more range.

Reassess and Repeat

We then palpate the area again, observing changes in taut fibers and tenderness. The decision of whether to repeat the cycle is based on how im-portant each muscle is in the overall treatment, as well as how much progress was made in the last cycle. If you feel that you're reaching a point of diminishing returns, this generally means you

Fig. 9-2. Treatment Cycle QR Code link-ing to video.

should attend to other muscles before continuing. Our protocols will guide you toward treating the functional antagonists—which can have an immediate beneficial effect—as well as the chain of satellite referral that might be setting the muscle up.

The CTB Treatment Cycle is the result of many years of clinical experience. Focusing on the shortening side first and providing feedback on agonist and antagonist during movement are critically important for convincing the nervous system to drop its protective engagement and allow tissues to return to normal length. We apply these principles to the treatment of every muscle, and we build our modules and protocols from these components.

The CTB Treatment Cycle is not only applicable to bodywork. We have great success using these same general principles in many settings, including self-care, yoga practice and adjustments, personal training, physical therapy, chiropractic, and more. The techniques change, but the treatment model is consistent.

The Proper Role of Stretching

After initial treatment, we do need to stretch muscles to return fibers to normal length and eliminate taut fibers. CTB uses stretching extensively after addressing any shortening dysfunction that might block the stretch. During any stretch, we must ask the patient what they're feeling. Dysfunction on the shortening side must be addressed first, as we have just described, or it could silently be blocking stretch of the antagonists. The client might feel nothing, or the stretch may seem to hit a hard end without a lot of discomfort. That generally indicates shortening dysfunction because the shortening muscle can silently send nociceptive signals that never rise above a threshold that triggers a conscious pain response.

If the client feels discomfort primarily on the stretching side, it indicates we are achieving a fiber length that is beginning to challenge the muscle's trigger points without being blocked on short, and we can continue the stretch. As more length is gained on the stretching side, the additional shortening in the antagonist could bring on shortening dysfunction, at which point we have to visit the other side of the joint. Increasing ROM in this way is a back-and-forth, iterative process. Ideally, compression can be maintained on both sides throughout treatment, but achieving this isn't always easy.

1. INCREMENTAL LENGTHENING DURING TREATMENT

CTB approaches stretching in increments. The first stage is lengthening fibers via movement combined with compression. We call this process working through range, and it is described below. Working through range changes the length of muscle fibers along with feedback being applied to both the stretch and the shortening side, which disrupts the tendency of the CNS to limit motion once a protective splinting has occurred.

2. LOCAL STRETCH: CONTRACT/RELAX

The second stage is designed to achieve length across the joints controlled by the muscle without involving a lot of other regional muscles. We generally focus on the joints directly influenced by the muscle. Local stretches are interleaved as part of the treatment cycle for each muscle.

We use neurological hacks—primarily MET, including contract/relax—with compressive or vibrational feedback on the stretching fibers to minimize protective resistance from the CNS. Applied to trigger point therapy, MET techniques provide an enhanced window for lengthening muscle fibers containing trigger points for a short time following active work. The stretch produces less referral, and the CNS allows the fibers to lengthen, unraveling the taut fibers.

We use contract/relax extensively in our work. Most often, we use the primary form: isometric contraction followed by stretch. We sometimes use the opposite: postisometric shortening. Making a muscle work, letting it relax, and then passively shortening it can work extremely well for muscles prone to contraction on short, such as the middle trapezius.

Contract/relax usually can generate significant additional pain-free ROM. It isn't unusual to see a 30 percent gain on a single repetition. In the CTB treatment cycle, we combine the stretch phase of contract/relax with therapeutic vibration on the stretching fibers as well as the referral zone. This process can be repeated several times, but more often, we intersperse contract/relax with the other phases of therapy, returning to it every few minutes.

In the contraction phase, we give the patient a touch cue that shows the patient the precise direction in which we want them to push to engage the muscle and ask the patient to press into our resistance. Higher levels of effort carry a greater risk of overload, and there is little benefit. We ask the patient to take a deep, diaphragmatic breath and hold it for five to thirty seconds as the muscle works, then we allow them to exhale and allow the muscle to fully relax. You can then move the muscle into stretch or shortening, noticing improved ROM.

It's essential to remember that each time you increase pain-free stretch ROM, you are increasing the shortening of the other side. Eventually, additional stretch may cause shortening dysfunction in the opposing muscles, at which point you must treat the shortening fibers or use a position that can address both simultaneously. The only way to discover this is by asking the patient to describe what they're feeling. Avoid questions like "How's the stretch?" or "How's the pressure?" because these constrain the answer.

3. REGIONAL STRETCH: RESOLVING STRETCH POSITIONS

We reserve larger, more comprehensive stretches for later in the treatment, after we have had the opportunity to work therapeutically with a wider set of muscles.

When I studied Thai massage, I learned many big, challenging stretches, some of which were supposed to be done early in the session. I learned quickly that these grand stretches had to be introduced very carefully, if at all, with my pain clients. With these individuals, it's important to restore length to individual muscles first and then select regional stretches that can be used for integration in some cases, but only if you fully understand the impact of each stretch. Thai massage has a large repertoire of stretch techniques, and during my years of experience teaching them, it was almost inevitable that someone would leave the mat with pain after certain stretch demonstrations. In addition, a full-body stretch involving many muscle groups is much harder to control.

To foster real change, the body needs an opportunity to integrate the therapeutic work applied to specific muscles, using its capacity for neuroplastic change to shift into a new normal across a broader range of muscle groups. That is why we do resolving stretches after the more specific work on a muscle group—or several. At that point, the quantum leaps in range and freedom can seem like magic, but that success is entirely dependent upon having done the detailed local work earlier in the session.

In Practice:
Thoracic Extension

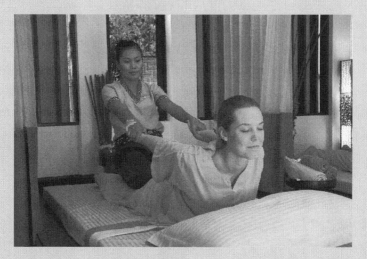

Fig. 9-3. Assisted cobra pose. The glutes are pinned by the therapist's knees as the lumbar spine is pulled into extension without compressive feedback on the spinal erectors. Creative Commons Attribution 2.0, Tara Angkor Hotel.

In the Thai massage kneeling cobra, the therapist kneels on the glutes to stabilize the pelvis and leans back while holding the client's wrists to bring them into an assisted, passive version of the yogic cobra backbend.

This is a very popular Thai massage pose—one that I was taught to perform routinely with every client before I learned trigger point therapy. It works well with flexible individuals who have a regular stretching practice and no spinal issues.

I began to encounter more and more clients and students who didn't do well with the pose and would get up with back pain. After I learned trigger point therapy and analyzed all of these poses from a functional anatomy perspective, I began to understand why. The client's weight hangs from the shoulders, and their pelvis is pinned by the therapist's body weight. Ideally, the back extension will be shared smoothly by all of the vertebrae, and no single area will encounter too much extension.

However, the reality is quite different among the general population. The lumbar vertebrae, unencumbered by the ribs, are able to extend in most people, even if they don't do backbends on a regular basis. Many individuals may already have excessive lordosis (extension) in their lumbar spine. The thoracic spine, however, could be stiff as a board and may even be locked in kyphosis (excessive flexion).

In a passive backbend like kneeling cobra, a stiff client's body will take the path of least resistance. The entire burden of extension will be absorbed in a few lumbar vertebrae, while the thoracic spine doesn't bend at all. This will force the lumbar spinal erectors abruptly into a shortened position, with no compression on those muscles or ability to guide the stretch into other parts of the spine. It may well produce a shortening activation as the lumbar spinal erectors contract on short and may extend some lumbar segments too abruptly, causing posterior disk compression.

Backbends are particularly problematic if they are done with no feedback on the spinal erectors. When people feel pain in a backbend, they don't generally feel it in the stretching muscles in the front of the body. They will feel a cramping in the back, which effectively limits the backbend and could activate continuing pain. The spinal erectors are particularly vulnerable to cramping on the short. For this reason, I eliminated backbends that fail to provide any compression on the spinal erectors as they are being asked to shorten.

In CTB, we use a much more therapeutic version of cobra, shown in Figure 9-4. In this version, the therapist sits on the high lumbar area rather than the pelvis, which provides excellent compressive feedback on the shortening spinal erectors, and also gives them a surface to curve gradually around rather than falling into an abrupt, hinge-like extension across a few vertebrae. The client's weight is close to the therapist's core, making it much easier for the therapist to control. The weight on the spinal erectors feels good and allows the client to relax without fear of cramping in the low back.

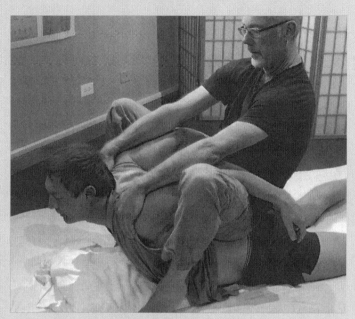

Fig. 9-4. Assisted cobra with compressive feedback on the lumbar spinal erectors from the therapist's sit bones. This is a much more therapeutic version that defeats contraction on short.

Even though the motion is similar, this modification allows the therapist to control the degree of compression and extension in each part of the spine, rather than leaving it to chance and letting the spine follow the path of least resistance. It can be an effective way to facilitate additional extension in the thoracic spine, which, being constrained by rib attachments, is much more difficult to mobilize. Through multiple cycles of contract/relax, this can facilitate real change and help undo the effects of a kyphotic, collapsed posture.

Larger stretches such as this sitting cobra are done later in the session to allow the CNS to integrate work across a number of muscle groups. We call these resolving stretches, as they are done with a specific goal of integrated movement across muscles that have already been worked on to some degree.

In Practice:
Resolving Stretch for Glutes and Low Back

Most lower body pain has some contribution from the gluteal muscles, quadratus lumborum, and adductors, so our Core Protocol for the Lower Body focuses treatment on these muscle groups. Low back pain also commonly has a gluteal component, along with shortening issues in the spinal erectors. After working all of these muscle groups, we use the cross-legged forward fold as a resolving stretch for all of these elements.

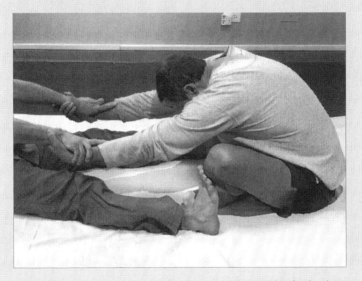

Fig. 9-5. Assisted forward fold, which integrates resolving stretches for the glutes and the back.

The client sits with crossed legs, to whatever extent they are comfortable. The pose works well with very limited clients who may not be comfortable sitting because we use contract/relax to quickly encourage the CNS to let go of its locked-in holding pattern in the glutes and low back. The client presses their feet down and knees up, which produces a medial rotation action in the hips, engaging the glutes strongly. Gluteus medius and minimus fibers convert to being 100 percent medial rotators once hip flexion reaches 90 degrees or more, and this external rotation in this position creates a strong gluteal stretch.

As the client presses their knees up, we ask them to arch their back—engaging both quadratus lumborum muscles as well as their spinal erectors—as the therapist provides resistance. We ask the client to hold their breath for five seconds, then have them relax and exhale; after a short pause, we use their arms to carry them forward. As they come into more hip and low back flexion and external rotation, they will feel the gluteal stretch. If they were limited, they might feel the stretch radiate down the legs and into the low back.

After a few seconds, we shorten the muscle slightly to take them off their new limit of comfortable stretch and repeat. This technique can provide a shocking level of release to someone who has become accustomed to constant pain and stiffness. I recall a student in a yoga class I taught who hadn't been able to sit comfortably or fold forward for years due to constant sciatic pain. Earlier in the class, we had done some work on her glutes. After this assisted stretch, she looked up with wide eyes, and then she looked over at her yoga teacher as tears rolled down her face.

"A story from one of my clients:

In the winter of 2019, I was attempting to do a "run streak" and was running at least a mile each day. In February, I, unfortunately, developed pretty severe hip pain, which ended the run streak. Not only that, but after about a week, it was nearly impossible to even walk. This was unlike any running injury that I'd experienced because it kept getting worse, and rest didn't seem to be helping. Reluctantly, I went to see a doctor for the pain. It was a sports med doctor, not just a general physician. I was diagnosed with hip bursitis, stretched for a brief time in the office, given paperwork with some stretches, and sent on my way with a prescription to stretch, take an OTC pain reliever and follow back to look at the possibility of a cortisone shot. I left the office bummed because I still could barely walk, and no way was I running.

Fortunately, I was referred by a friend to Stacey Styborski. When I first went to see Stacey, I was hesitant as I didn't know what to expect. I just knew that a "massage" was not going to get the job done. I was pleasantly surprised! The dialogue to determine not only where the pain was located but what was causing it was amazing. I was blown away that for hip pain, she knew just where to focus on other parts of my body to help with the pain. Within a few visits, I was running again!

The ability to find the trigger points in my body to help with pain all over is fascinating. The knowledge in her CTB approach of how the various muscles work to trigger other parts of the body and healing or stretching them is amazing. The combination of stretches, maneuvering, and stimulation to adjust my body works so much better than anything I've experienced. The most comforting part of my visits is that I've never gotten a suggestion for any sort of medication. Nor has there ever been anything other than, "We can work to get this better."

"When she first came to me, she could hardly move. I did the CTB Core Lower Body Protocol with her—very carefully at first. She got relief from that work, and her gluteal muscles were very troubled due to being a hyperpronator and having a leg length discrepancy. She now wears corrective insoles and a heel lift, and is fully able to run again."
—Stacey Styborski, CTB practitioner, Ohio

CHAPTER 10

Coaching the Body Bodywork Techniques

I feel that many bodyworkers place too much emphasis on tricks and techniques without understanding why and when they should be used or how those tricks and techniques affect muscles and joints. That said, my team and I have compiled a powerful library of techniques that I've spent years analyzing and refining to find the best approach for each muscle. The key to appropriate use of techniques is having a framework for assessment and analysis that uncovers the true source of dysfunction and guides us to work on muscles in the correct order. That's the purpose of the CTB protocols.

In this section, I'll present a sampling of useful techniques that we've developed over the years, with an in-depth description of muscular and therapeutic effects. While we don't have room in this book to fully catalogue our technique repertoire, I hope that this chapter will provide some ideas for how to incorporate the CTB approach into your own work. I've selected these particular techniques because they are some of the most important and useful, and they exemplify how we've adapted some traditional Thai techniques for use as highly efficient means of doing trigger point therapy on specific muscles and their antagonists.

I have several important criteria in selecting and designing techniques, whether they are intended for bodywork or self-care:

Design Criteria for Techniques

Moving the body—your own or someone else's—can be a lot of work, and it can be hard on the therapist if they rely too much on peripheral strength. It's paramount that the therapist use techniques meant to avoid or prevent injury to their own bodies.

I teach a lot of massage therapists at my school, and many of them show substantial wear and tear on their bodies, even if they haven't been working for long. Some of this is due to the philosophy and intent behind the techniques. For example, if you think what you're doing is crushing and breaking up adhesions and scar tissue, then strength and force seem valuable. But taut fibers aren't scar tissue, and excessive force invokes the body's protective response and inevitably has a negative impact on the therapist's hands, arms, and shoulders. Excessive use of pressure and strength can also produce a danger response in the CNS because it feels invasive and unstable, causing it to invoke its protective splinting engagement of the very muscles you're attempting to treat.

My martial arts background has informed my approach to body mechanics and movement. While strength is an advantage, the best martial artists don't tend to be the strongest. In fact, balance, leverage, and moving energy from the core to the periphery are far more important than raw strength. I strongly emphasize bodywork techniques that keep the work close to the practitioner's core and allow them to use their body weight as opposed to peripheral strength.

CTB uses compression, but we almost always pair it with some kind of movement, which presents its own challenges. We often hold compression or vibration while the fibers are moving, which also serves to invoke neuroplastic change in the CNS. This is far more effective than held static compression, but the therapist needs to ensure that they are moving their client's body and compressing the target muscles without causing stress to their own body, particularly their shoulders.

Massage therapists sometimes use stripping and cross-fiber techniques with the elbow held away from the body, which places extreme stress on the therapist's shoulder. We most often reverse this approach, holding an area of compression or vibration while the muscle length changes. We position the client's body so that both the compression and the muscle movement happen via a simple shift in the therapist's body weight. It's far easier to use body weight without stress on the shoulders when the work is very close to your core. We keep the area where we're applying compression close to the therapist's body. I call it the principle of Working From Ease.

There are important reasons not to work with stress and tension beyond the obvious benefits for the therapist. As you move contact away from your core and into your periphery, your touch will convey more of a struggle, less stability, and more effort to your client. A large part of our therapeutic goal is helping the client's CNS to downregulate and drop protection, but if the client senses that the therapist is using all of their strength and has poor control, the CNS is less likely to feel safe and let go. In addition, if the therapist is struggling, they'll be less able to sense small changes in tissue and the CNS response in their client. It's a win for everyone to work with as much ease as possible.[36]

---

36 Thai techniques can be wonderful in this way, but you have to pay close attention to how you set up your body position, or the benefits will not be seen. The Thai repertoire makes extensive use of feet, knees, shins, even sitting compression. I offer a very popular course on Hands-Free Thai techniques in my curriculum, where we explore this approach to working from ease in detail. Again, these techniques have major benefits for both client and therapist. Broad points of contact, plus the stability of body weight as opposed to shaky muscular strength provide a safer, less threatening environment for the client's CNS to accept the pressure and reduce protective control.

Changing Fiber Length with Compression

I've stated how important movement is in rehabilitating tissues that have become locked down with taut fibers. We rarely use techniques that only allow for compression without movement. I look for techniques that allow for changing fiber length while treating the trigger point area with compression or vibration. Conversely, we make limited use of stretches that don't allow for feedback on the lengthening or the shortening fibers, with the exception of resolving stretches, which are only used after fibers on both sides of the joint have been treated.

Working Fibers into Short

In most muscles, the first step of the treatment cycle is to work the muscle into short with compression or vibration. We need to apply increasing pressure as the fibers get shorter, ideally using our body weight. Without some form of feedback in the shortening muscle, the fibers may contract painfully on the short, which is therapeutically counterproductive.

Working Both Sides of the Joint

I place high value on techniques that easily allow some manner of feedback on agonist and antagonist during movement, without the therapist having to change positions. This increases our opportunity to significantly expand pain-free ROM, downregulating the CNS as it witnesses the expanded range without discomfort.

In the next sections, I'll go into detail about how to apply a sampling of our techniques and also where their use is most appropriate.

Kneeling Under the Calf

DESCRIPTION

We use this particular technique—one in a category we call sitting under the leg—to work the tibialis anterior/soleus combination. These muscles can cause pain in the calf, Achilles tendon, heel, front of the ankle, and big toe, as well as being primary suspects in clients with ankle rigidity.

The therapist's folded leg serves as a firm support and compresses the soleus/gastrocnemius as the therapist's body weight compresses the tibialis anterior from above. The firm compression on both sides of the joint is helpful to facilitate fast change.

MUSCLES

Treated muscles include tibialis anterior, soleus, gastrocnemius, and extensor digitorum longus, all into length and into short.

SETUP

Kneel with your proximal leg under the client's mid-calf, with the client's leg close to your body. Palpate the fibers of the tibialis anterior belly for tautness and tenderness, and position your ulnar ridge (not your elbow) directly over that area. Take care to avoid compression directly on the tibia.

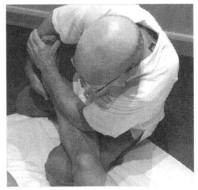
Fig. 10-1. Working tibialis anterior into short.

To work into short, place the ball of the client's foot just below your elbow crease, clasp your hands together to form a stable structure, and lean toward the client's head to transfer weight into the forearm compression of the belly of the muscle. Move slightly and repeat several times. Observe if the tibialis anterior tendon engages as you dorsiflex the foot. This indicates contraction on the short. Use more body weight and less dorsiflexion if contracting on short, attempting to minimize the tendon engagement. This

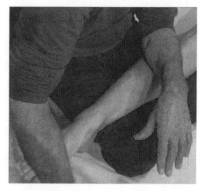

Fig. 10-2. Tibialis anterior into stretch, shortening the soleus.

action retrains the muscle to shorten more gracefully. Compression treatment of the tibialis anterior followed by contract/relax will improve contraction on short.

CONTRACT/RELAX

Place your distal forearm on the top of the client's forefoot and have them press up into your resistance. Have them inhale and hold for five seconds. On exhale, press down with both forearms to plantar flex the foot and work the tibialis anterior into length, shortening the soleus. Be cautious because the pressure on the shortened soleus could be very tender. Return to work into short, and observe any improvement in taut fibers, tenderness, and contraction on short.

VARIATIONS

Use vibration on the tibialis anterior through its entire range. Vibration works extremely well on the dense tibialis anterior fibers. EPS is effective to downregulate hypersensitivity on either tibialis anterior or soleus.

The Crossover Stretch

DESCRIPTION

We use this adduction stretch for the gluteal fibers and TFL to reveal any referral from those muscles that might normally be dormant at rest. The crossover stretch is very useful as an assessment early in the session.

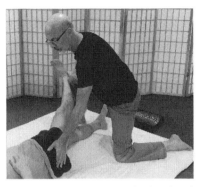

Fig. 10-3. Crossover stretch for the gluteal abductor fibers.

Later in the session, this technique can also be used as a resolving stretch for gluteal work.

Clients with a sciatica diagnosis may have a belief that the sciatic nerve is being impinged at the spine. This stretch vividly demonstrates that by simply stretching the gluteal fibers, we can reproduce their pain, thereby establishing a powerful body anchor for the origins of their radiating hip and leg pain.

MUSCLES

This stretch works gluteus medius, gluteus minimus, and TFL. Dropping the leg closer to the mat emphasizes the anterior gluteal fibers and TFL. Raising it higher focuses it on the posterior gluteal fibers. As the gluteal fibers stretch, this pose shortens adductor longus and may cause groin pain due to contraction on short.

SETUP

Lunge with your foot placed on the other side of the client's far leg. Grasp the foot of the near leg at the heel and support your arm with your own leg. Your body and lunge should do the work of moving the client's leg. As you lunge forward, monitor for any resistance or discomfort. Referral starting in the hip and radiating down the leg indicates that the gluteus/QL complex is generating a radiating sciatic pattern.

CONTRACT/RELAX

Have the client abduct their leg laterally into your resistance, hold for a five count with inhale, and slowly move into stretch by lunging across after they exhale.

VARIATIONS

The degree of hip flexion determines which gluteal fibers are emphasized in the stretch. Position the foot closer to the mat in front of your shin to focus on the anterior glutes and TFL. Your hand at the top of the leg stabilizes the hip and prevents it from floating up above the mat, which would lose some of the adduction in favor of hip flexion. Vibration can be used on the gluteal fibers to increase stretch if the technique isn't being used as an assessment.

Adductor Variations: Adductor Longus
DESCRIPTION

For therapists using their hands, the large leg muscles can be particularly challenging. In addition, focused techniques that address a single muscle are not very effective due to the key functional relationships between the adductors and the glutes.

To work with these muscles without putting strain on our own bodies, we use a powerful series of technique variations derived from traditional Thai bodywork poses, as well as my background in martial arts. Here, we apply what we call HandsFree Thai techniques, which tend to employ broad compression and body weight and can provide powerful depth with ease. In these approaches, in particular, it's key that we keep work close to the core, rely upon leverage, and use broad, deep compression with lots of distraction. When we do, our client's CNS is much more able to let go, and when combined with therapeutic vibration and working both sides of the joint, these techniques can be magically effective. The idea is to position your body so a slight change in body weight can do a substantial amount of therapeutic work.

We can work the adductor longus into short, neutral, and various degrees of stretch with very little change in body position.

The variations described here allow the therapist to work the adductors into short, into length, and various degrees of external rotation. The latter action lengthens both the adductors and the posterior gluteus fibers, a double action that can help normalize that important relationship.

MUSCLES

Gluteus medius and minimus, piriformis, adductor longus, and adductor magnus.

SETUP

Variation A: Come into a low lunge with your inside sit bone resting on your raised heel, perched on the ball of your foot. Your other knee should be on the ground, abducted enough so you clear the client's knee. Tuck the client's ankle tightly against your ASIS, and slide in close enough to their leg so your

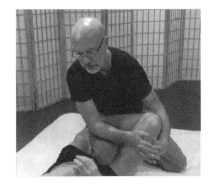

Fig. 10-5. Variation B: Working adductor longus into short

knee comes through and your shin is over their adductor longus fibers. Rest your inside arm on your own leg. When set up properly, you should be able to fold forward very slightly and have the compression on the adductor longus increase substantially as stretch is also increased.

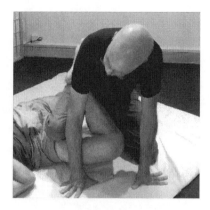

Variation B: Clasp your hands around the client's knee and lean back to pull their adductor longus fibers into your shin or knee. As the client's leg adducts, the adductor longus fibers will shorten, and you can adjust the position of your knee or shin to target a specific area.

Fig. 10-6. Variation C: Adding external rotation stretch to adductors and glutes.

Variation C: This adds external rotation at the hip. Variation C can be done with or without contract/relax. Brace your hands on the mat to stabilize the client's leg so it doesn't move into hip flexion as you come up. Lift your hips, which will lift the client's ankle and externally rotate the femur at the hip. At 90 degrees of hip flexion, all of the gluteus medius and minimus fibers become medial rotators, which is a shared action with adductor longus and magnus.

This technique exploits that shared action to provide a stretch in the glutes and the adductors at the same time. This can be very effective after you've done some initial treatment on both muscle groups, and sometimes it's most useful to do this variation late in the session for clients with severe glute/adductor issues.

Fig. 10-7. Adductor variations QR code.

CONTRACT/RELAX

Have the client lift their knee into your resistance. You can also have them press their ankle down into your leg, which will add an element of medial rotation along with the adduction. On exhale, lean forward, optionally raising your hips in Variation C.

Scapular Assessment and Cleaning the Wing
DESCRIPTION

Our scapular positioning module begins with an assessment of scapular position and motion, along with assessment and treatment of muscles that may be contracting on the short. We begin moving the scapula very slowly and gently clockwise and counterclockwise, paying close attention to any points in the motion that are limited and sticky or where the scapula seems to suddenly jump to a new position. The latter may seem as if the client is consciously taking over active control, but in

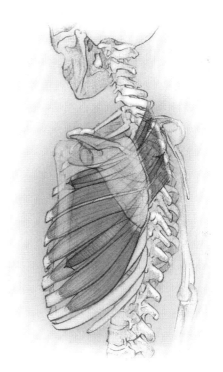

Fig. 10-8. The fiber direction of scapular muscles determines the direction of pull.

most cases, it's due to certain fibers contracting as they shorten and is not voluntary. This is an excellent diagnostic for which specific fibers are problematic. For example, if the scapula suddenly adducts and elevates on its own as we circle closer to the spine, this is an indication that the rhomboids are contracting on short.

Cleaning the wing is derived from a traditional shiatsu and Thai technique, in which the client's fingers or thumb are used as a stationary point of compression as the scapula is adducted. The idea is that the

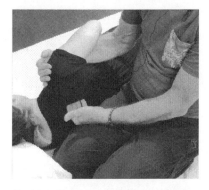

Fig. 10-9. Cleaning the Wing with fingertips braced on your leg.

scapula should smoothly slide over the client's fingers, but it's common for the trapezius and rhomboid fibers to harden and contract as they shorten, so the muscle then feels like a wall that the therapist's fingers cannot penetrate. If the scapula is abducted enough, the fibers will lengthen and soften. This makes it possible to see exactly where the fibers begin to contract. If the fingers are then stabilized at that point as the scapula is adducted, we can use the firm compression to turn off the contraction on short response, which is extremely helpful in normalizing scapular motion.

You will very often find that the muscles medial to the scapular border are intransigent and difficult to soften. Therapists tend to waste a lot of time in this area because they don't understand the neurological relationships involved. There are antagonistic fibers in the serratus anterior for each of the fiber directions in the medial muscles, and those must be treated before the body will allow the adductive fibers to soften. The power of the scapular positioning module comes from how we always work directly opposed fibers in the serratus anterior and other antagonists as we work the scapular adductor fibers.

MUSCLES
Middle and low trapezius and rhomboids.

SETUP
Kneel parallel to the client's back with their scapula just in front of your abdomen. You need to be close enough to the client's back so your leg can serve as a platform for your hand; you cannot do this properly with your hand floating in the air. The idea is to stabilize your hand so that it is a fixed point of resistance. You then

Fig. 10-10. Cleaning the Wing example video QR code.

bring the scapula to your fingers or thumb by leaning away from the client. Monitor the state of the mid trapezius and rhomboid muscles as you begin to adduct the scapula. If contracting on the short, you need to have your fingers meet the scapula prior to the point at which they harden. Keep your fingers or thumb rigid and begin to bring the scapula toward your hand. If you are meeting a hard wall, adjust your position so you contact the scapula with it farther away from the spine.

The goal is to allow your fingers to wrap the muscles around and underneath the scapula just prior to contraction on short. Some preliminary softening with vibration is very helpful, and if you struggle to get underneath the scapula, you will most likely need to do some serratus anterior treatment first.

CONTRACT/RELAX
You can gain some immediate improvement by placing your hand on the client's scapula and having them push their shoulder back into your pressure. Hold for five seconds or more, and on exhale, go back into the technique. Note that this is a form of contract/

relax in which we shorten after the effort rather than stretch—this variation can be used in most muscles but is particularly effective here and with muscles that tend to contract on short.

After you can consistently let the scapula slide over your fingers, have the client take a deep breath, and on exhale, hook the scapula with your fingers and lean back so the scapula strongly abducts. This can create more space in the shoulder for clients whose scapula has chronically pulled in toward the neck.[37]

Serratus Anterior Techniques
DESCRIPTION

Serratus anterior is a somewhat difficult muscle to treat, and it is poorly understood by many bodyworkers. The fibers may feel thin and hard and difficult to distinguish from rib bodies. It's a very broad muscle with many distinct serrations, comprising a wide range of fiber directions. The more superior fibers range from difficult to access to inaccessible.

That said, the serratus anterior is an essential muscle in the CTB system. We treat it as the primary scapular protractor and antagonist to mid/low trapezius and rhomboids.

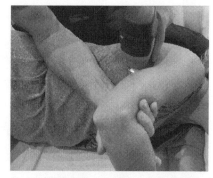

On most people, the lowest fiber attaches to the ninth rib, but there is some variation, and on some individuals, attachments may extend to the twelfth rib. It must be treated with sensitivity and a lot of scapular movement. When arm motion is limited, the serratus

Fig. 10-11. Kneeling alongside the client allows the therapist to manage the arm and the tool while keeping the work close to their body.

_____

37 The clavicular pectoralis major is often a contributor to this sort of narrowing.

anterior is likely involved due to its key role in stabilization as the scapula rotates. Due to the close functional and neurological relationship between opposing fibers, we must treat the trapezius, rhomboids, and serratus anterior as a unit.

We start by treating the serratus in a more shortened position. A shortened resting length is generally the default condition of the muscle in someone with shoulder pain. Their scapula will be protracted, meaning the serratus fibers are already shorter than normal. You can shorten the serratus anterior by draping the arm forward so that it carries the scapula forward.

Vibration is ideal and much preferred to pure bodywork, which requires a great degree of sensitivity and skill pressing on the side of the ribs since they are sensitive on most people anyway. Bodywork also lacks the beneficial distractive effect of the vibration. We use the soft tip with the Muscle Liberator to provide a more gentle percussion in the serratus anterior, whose trigger point areas can be quite sensitive because of their location on the ribs. Once the muscle softens a bit, try to localize trigger point areas based on their hardness using gentle cross-fiber palpation.

There are two primary bundles of fibers that radiate out from the inferior angle and the superior medial border. The latter is rather inaccessible until the fibers cross into the superior axilla, but take care to avoid the structures of the brachial plexus. Move the Muscle Liberator in an arc near the inferior angle and lateral border of the scapula, from the lowest fiber bundle (which generally attaches to the ninth rib) to the area under the arm toward the shoulder joint. Always direct the tool toward the ribs rather than the soft tissue of the axilla.

As you use the vibration or compression, introduce some arm movement. You should assess scapular rotation prior to beginning treatment, and it will usually exhibit some limitation. Rotation should dramatically improve once you've done some treatment on related mid-trapezius/rhomboid and serratus fibers, including contract/relax.

MUSCLES
Serratus anterior.

SETUP
Position yourself close to the client, either kneeling parallel or facing the client's back, or both. You will need to use body weight to apply manual compression. The Muscle Liberator does not require use of body weight and generally should be held close to your body. Find the best position that allows you to comfortably manage the arm at the same time as you apply compression or vibration.

CONTRACT/RELAX

To contract, have the client inhale and thrust their entire shoulder forward into your fore-arm resistance, which engages the entire muscle. Upon exhale, use your arm to adduct the scapula toward the spine as you apply vibration or compression.

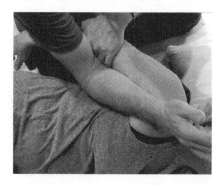

Fig. 10-12. Client projects their shoulder forward against your resistance. On exhale press the elbow back to retract the scapula for a serratus stretch.

Be attentive to any discomfort or pinching between the scapula and the spine, as this could be due to the mid trapezius and rhomboids contracting on short. If this happens, it will produce a hard limit on the serratus stretch, and you will need to treat those muscles more thoroughly before you can complete your work on serratus anterior. It's quite common and useful to move back and forth between agonist and antagonist a few times.

It can also be very helpful when attempting to restore scapular rotation to do contract/relax with arm flexion or abduction and adduct on stretch with the scapula. The serratus/trapezius/rhomboid trio is heavily involved in scapular rotation. The scapula must rotate during arm movements, and these muscles must collaborate properly for full range of arm movement without pain. Retraining this neurological relationship is critical, which is why we always treat serratus anterior, trapezius, and rhomboids as part of the same module in our Core Upper Body Protocol.

Half Cobra with Feet: Resolving Stretch
DESCRIPTION

After working on the core shoulder muscles, we use a technique that combines arm extension, scapular retraction, spinal extension and rotation, and external rotation of the arm to reset the scapular positioning muscles. This pose is ideal because it lengthens the muscles that have a tendency to shorten and pull the scapula into protraction while providing compressive feedback on the problematic posterior muscles that tend to contract on the short. A pure stretch without that feedback doesn't fully support the CNS in moving past its dysfunctional patterns. Even subtle contraction on short in the iliocostalis, trapezius, and rhomboids can defeat the stretch of the serratus anterior, pectoralis major, and pectoralis minor. Iliocostalis is an important muscle for shoulder pain, as it is sensitive to leg length discrepancy and can initiate satellite referral into the shoulder muscles.

The technique begins by holding the arm loosely and using the heel along the spinal erectors to soften them. Working with the heel along the iliocostalis and longissimus, let the client roll forward a bit with each press, and then gently pull the arm back as you release. This creates a rocking motion that prepares the muscles for the deeper stretches that follow. Make a few passes up and down the high side of the spine, and then place the heel in the high lumbar, have the client take a deep breath, and, on exhale, press your foot in a bit more and rock back to create a twisting motion in the spine along with extension of the shoulder away from the mat. Since the net effect is extending and rotating one side of the spine, we classify this pose as a half cobra, named for the prone yoga backbend.

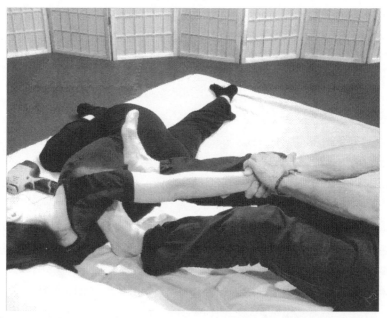

Fig. 10-13. Half Cobra with Feet. Lean back, pinning a point on the spinal erectors with your heel, causing spinal rotation.

It is helpful to press with the foot slightly before you lean back. Otherwise, the client may find the action confusing and resist. The heel pressure is important and provides a fulcrum point around which the spine bends as well as providing feedback to the spinal erectors to minimize contraction as they shorten. Every client will have different challenges, and you need to honor their limitations. Some may find the arm extension difficult, in which case you need to adjust your position so as not to force too much stretch on the pectoralis major and minor and biceps. The arm can bend, and you can hold it in the upper arm for more control and gentler arm extension.

Move your heel closer to the scapula and repeat, and continue for a few repetitions with your foot in different positions. A second phase can then be added, in which you use your other foot to essentially do the cleaning the wing technique. Some clients may feel distress as the scapula adducts, so feedback on the mid trapezius and rhomboids is needed to defeat contraction on short. Push the arm forward a bit, pushing the scapula into protraction, and place your foot flat against the client's back with your toes near the medial border. On exhale, allow the scapula to ride up over your foot if possible. If there is still active contraction happening in the trapezius, this will be difficult or impossible, but sometimes it can provide the final degree of release in the shoulder. This is a powerful combination, and you can do both feet together, with your heel compressing the erectors as your other foot compresses the medial scapular muscles.

Use caution with this technique in the beginning of the treatment, and don't attempt to push the patient beyond their capacity. It can be difficult to get right. Work slowly and with the breath. It can help to do a contract/relax on each repetition.

MUSCLES

All scapular positioning muscles, including trapezius, rhomboids, serratus anterior, pectoralis minor, pectoralis major, levator scapulae, in addition to rotator cuff muscles, spinal erectors, such as longissimus, and iliocostalis.

SETUP

You should set yourself up so that rather than being at 90 degrees from the client's back, you reduce the angle by moving closer to the client's feet. This will reduce the amount of arm extension needed in the full stretch, which is important until you trust the client's ability to extend at the shoulder. Be close enough to their back so that your leg just straightens in the full stretch. Hold at the wrist and forearm unless this presents too much challenge in arm extension. You can reduce the challenge by moving closer and letting the arm bend, holding above the elbow. Externally rotating the arm will greatly increase the challenge on pectoralis major, so be attentive and check in with the client.

CONTRACT/RELAX

You can use contract/relax on the first couple of repetitions or on every repetition to maximize ease and benefit for the client. Set up for the stretch and have the client take a deep breath and pull their arm and shoulder forward as you resist. This will engage all of the anterior muscles—serratus anterior, clavicular pectoralis major, and pectoralis minor—making it much easier for the client to let go into the stretch.

"Lucinda is serious about riding horses and has had several falls. This is her description of her symptoms from her most recent and serious fall:

My injury was caused when, while galloping on my horse, he fell to his knees, and I flew like a yard dart, head first. I did not have ANY bruises from the fall. I was knocked unconscious for about thirty seconds before coming to. I went to the ER, where they did X-rays and a CAT scan, which didn't show anything. They told me to follow up with my doctor and to take it easy for a few days.

Went to see my MD the following week. Told him about my severe migraines, light sensitivity, and fatigue. He took more X-rays and told me to go home and take it easy and that I should be recovered in a couple of weeks.

My symptoms included SEVERE MIGRAINES, occipital neuralgia, whiplash, extreme fatigue, light sensitivity, sound sensitivity, dizziness, and confusion.

A good friend, Jill Duncan, reached out to me (after seeing some posts on Facebook) because she was confident she could help me cure the migraines, and she did! It took five to six visits over a two to three month period, but they are 95 percent GONE! For months PRIOR to seeing her, I'd take four ibuprofen and two Tylenol for my migraines with only minor change. When seeing Jill, I switched to CBD oil (with little to no THC), and my migraines would go from a nine or ten to a one because of the work she did. She basically dismantled the pieces of the migraine. Currently, I have to watch my posture and keep up with trigger point therapy when symptoms creep up.

I am so incredibly grateful to Jill for reaching out to me and helping me heal.

"My assessments showed Lucinda to be an extreme hyperpronator, and she also carried a head-forward posture most of the time due to both the postural collapse from hyperpronation and her job as a graphic designer with poor workstation ergonomics. I fit her with Hyperpronation Correction Insoles. She came to me with severe suboccipital pain on both sides, severe pain shooting through to her right eye, and nausea when flexing or extending her neck.

"I did a CTB Shoulder, Head, and Neck Protocol in her first session and found that she had trigger point issues in her low trapezius that were referring up into her mid and high trapezius, and her right splenius cervicis was causing the pain she reported at C7 as well as her eye pain. The migraines decreased dramatically. Over a few more sessions, we worked with her posterior cervical muscles, SCMs (which were likely triggering the nausea), and levator scapulae and scalenes, which had been causing pain between her shoulder blades for many years.

"While she had the falls and those triggered acute events, her overall vulnerability was set up by years of head-forward posture and scapular positioning issues, creating a situation that was ripe for problems after she had a fall. Once her neck and shoulder muscles could be in a more balanced state, she has been clear of serious issues for an extended time."

—Jill Duncan, CTB master practitioner and instructor,
St. Louis, Missouri

CHAPTER 11

Using Tools with CTB

I take a practical approach to the use of tools in the CTB system. Through my many years of experimenting and developing Coaching the Body, some tools have been extraordinarily successful, so I kept them. Others didn't seem to enhance my work, so I don't use them. I use what works. My sole criterion is whether the tool adds something in terms of effectiveness, speed, or both. The ones I find most valuable are therapeutic vibration and percussion tools—so much so that I developed my own, the Muscle Liberator—and electronic point stimulation or EPS.

No tool is a magic bullet or panacea; effectiveness in CTB comes from understanding, not from a particular tool or technique. That being said, I have found that certain muscles respond much more quickly and thoroughly when I use the EPS or Muscle Liberator as compared to straight manual therapy. These are the primary tools that I've found to be useful, and I'm certain that more will be discovered as we continue to develop this modality.

Therapeutic Vibration Tools

The concept of using percussion/vibration on the body has been an ongoing subject of medical experimentation since the late 1800s. So-called "massage guns" are widely available today, but there has been little true understanding of why they might be effective.

When we began our own experiments in applying these tools to trigger point therapy, we found that while the effects were promising, the combination of head design, frequency, and percussion amplitude in existing tools left something to be desired for our purposes. We took on the task of designing our own tool and heads several years ago, and the result was the Muscle Liberator. In the intervening years, this tool has

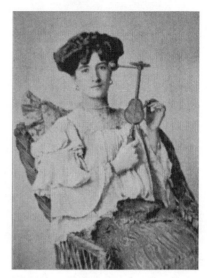

Fig. 11-1. A nineteenth-century experiment in using hand-operated percussion to relieve headaches.

become an essential component of our system due to its phenomenal ability to provide distraction and micro-stretch on individually targeted fiber bundles.

As always, the tool is only as good as the knowledge of its operator. The next section will introduce background regarding why percussion is valuable in releasing trigger points, as well as our specific design goals when we created the Muscle Liberator.

THE PHYSIOLOGY OF PERCUSSION

Percussion appeared in the original *Lower Extremities* volume of the Travell and Simons *Trigger Point Manual*.[38] The technique, called Percussion and Stretch, involved bringing a muscle to its stretch barrier and using a rubber mallet to repeatedly strike the trigger point in the same place. Dr. Travell particularly liked using it in the quadratus lumborum, saying, "This apparently simple

---

38 J. G. Travell and Simons *Lower Extremity* volume, 1992, 10.

technique can be remarkably effective." Even so, she never fully explored the technique. Percussion also shows up in the traditional Thai repertoire and other Asian modalities, where muscles are routinely percussed under stretch with a loose fist, side of the hand, or other techniques. Interestingly, there is another traditional Thai technique, called jap sen, that involves strong snapping palpation with the thumbs. The goal is jumping engagement of the muscle fibers, which is considered a therapeutic result. In trigger point therapy as well, repeated production of twitch responses in fibers is known to soften taut fibers.

Percussing a muscle can have powerful healing effects. When a muscle fiber is placed under stretch and tapped with a soft mallet or hand, a momentary micro-stretch occurs in those fibers as they bend and release, not unlike what happens when a guitar string is plucked. Following the distortion of the fibers, they show a spike of engagement, and it has long been speculated that this is due to a reflex response from the muscle spindles sending a signal to the spinal cord, which then causes a reflex activation of the muscle.

However, just banging on a muscle won't treat the pain or remap the CNS. Resistance to stretch is built into human muscular physiology. The myotatic reflex is a normal response to muscle stretch, in which organs embedded into muscle fibers, called spindles, send a signal to the spinal cord and cause a reflex return of motor engagement, which causes the muscle to resist the stretch. This arrangement is necessary for safe and smooth motion. Uncontrolled stretching would be dangerous and spasmodic. If the muscle also has taut fibers due to trigger points, another protective mechanism comes into play that increases resistance dramatically.

When a muscle containing a taut fiber is stretched, the nociceptive stream from the stretched trigger point will increase. The brain then receives an "injury" danger signal from the periphery and bases its response on how long the situation has gone on, how upregulated the system is, and consequently, how likely it is to generate pain. Over time, sensitivity increases, and in tandem, the CNS is more likely to splint or send an engagement signal to the muscle. The more pain is produced, the more protective engagement will result, inhibiting the stretch. An extreme case of this can be seen in advanced shoulder pain patients, in which the therapist even reaching for the arm to move it can trigger painful wincing, in keeping with Moseley's associative pain memory model.[39] A vivid memory of the pain on stretch can actually trigger the pain again. It's virtually impossible to stretch that patient's shoulder muscles without utilizing some neurological hacks that interfere with the memorized pain response that their CNS has fallen into.

A study by Alberto Botter and his colleagues found that when a muscle is percussed, there is a measurable engagement that is confined to the tapped muscle fibers, and the intensity radiates out from the site of the tap.[40] This important discovery demonstrates that the muscle's firing is not due to a reflex response but originates within the fibers themselves. In contrast, when the doctor taps your knee and your leg moves, it's due to a neurological reflex response to the tendon suddenly being stretched. Reflexes involve sending a signal upstream to the spinal cord, which the CNS then processes, and a motor signal being sent back to the muscle, creating a built-in transmission delay. The sort of engagement observed by Botter is quite different. There is no round trip to the spinal cord but rather a virtually immediate contractile response that

---

39 Lorimer G. Moseley and Johan W. S. Vlaeyen, "Beyond Nociception: The Imprecision Hypothesis of Chronic Pain," *Pain* 156, no. 1 (2015): 35–38, http://dx.doi.org/10.1016/j.pain.0000000000000014.

40 Alberto Botter, Taian M. Vieira, Tommaso Geri, and Silvestro Roatta, "The Peripheral Origin of Tap-induced Muscle Contraction Revealed by Multi-Electrode Surface Electromyography in Human Vastus Medialis," *Scientific Reports* 10, no. 1 (2020): 1–11, doi:10.1038/s41598-020-59122-z.

originates exactly where the muscle fiber was struck, triggered by the sudden stretch of the sarcomeres. In addition, this study found that the contraction is confined to the particular fiber bundle that was struck, as opposed to a reflex, which fires the entire muscle.

Botter's study is highly relevant to trigger point therapy, although it wasn't conducted with that in mind. In trigger point therapy, we make use of a phenomenon known as the local twitch response (LTR). When snapping palpation or needling is used on fibers containing trigger points, the fibers will show this same spike of engagement. The twitch response is considered a confirmative finding for trigger points, and based on the results of the Botter study, it may be a greatly amplified version of something that happens in normal muscle tissue as well. This would indicate that the nociceptive chemical milieu of the trigger point adds fuel to the mechanism of firing the fiber after it has been suddenly deformed. We exploit this characteristic in how we use our percussion tool, the Muscle Liberator.

A PERCUSSION TOOL FOR TRIGGER POINT WORK

I mentioned earlier the importance of distraction to the CTB methodology and to trigger point work in general, and two of the most important elements of distraction are vibration and percussion. To that end, I developed a tool called the Muscle Liberator, which has made many people aware of CTB. Treating someone with

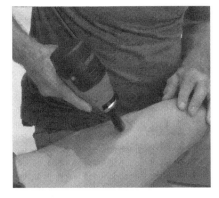

Fig. 11-2. Applying vibration to vastus medialis with the Muscle Liberator.

what looks like a power drill certainly gets people's attention.

People tend to have a variety of uninformed but strong reactions to my Muscle Liberator videos. Some love them, saying that it looks fantastic and that they want to use it on their shoulders where it hurts. Others comment that there is no substitute for the hands and human touch when doing massage. They claim you can't feel what's happening with the tissues. And others say that it looks incredibly painful or that it's a gimmick. I see things differently.

While I'm excited about the results we get with this tool within the CTB system, there is a lot of general misunderstanding regarding the use of vibration and percussion tools.

We designed the Muscle Liberator heads with a fine tip to localize the percussion to specific fibers. Other tools on the market are sold with much larger heads, usually quite hard. This makes it impossible to target specific fibers and has the potential to injure bony landmarks such as the spine.

We cast the Muscle Liberator heads out of forgiving silicone, with narrow tips and varying degrees of firmness and elasticity so they can be used on specific fibers near bony surfaces. The pressure we use is relatively light, and the goal is to provide micro stretches and vibratory distraction as hacks to get the CNS to release taut fibers. We aren't ironing out entire muscles; we're targeting specific fiber bundles with taut fibers.

The tool has a variable speed trigger, allowing the operator to smoothly change the percussion rate from 0 to 2,400 strokes per minute. One of our primary goals with the tool and head combination was to construct an assistive device for trigger point therapy that would simulate the fiber snapping/twitch response procedure but at a higher rate than is possible with hands alone. Our original design goals have been met very successfully. As you move the head from fiber to fiber, you can notice the specific twitch responses in each fiber rippling through the muscle.

In the case of targeted fiber percussion with the Muscle Liberator, the fiber lengthening and returning to normal happens so quickly that there isn't enough time for the nociceptive input to be processed by the CNS and rise above the threshold to be interpreted as pain. It's a hack for teasing the taut fiber into more length before the pain response can even kick in. As Travell did with her hammer, we bring the muscle to its stretch barrier and then use the percussion to move through the barrier.

If you use the Muscle Liberator in the shoulder, the vibration will shake the entire area and effectively mask most other pain. Without painful feedback upon movement, the CNS allows painfully contracted taut fibers to lengthen and allows for a new experience of pain-free movement.

I've found that the rapid-fire percussion from the Muscle Liberator also creates a tremendous amount of neurological distraction, providing the benefits of the spray and stretch technique mentioned in Chapter 6 without the downside of consuming an expensive, nonrenewable product that must be applied to the skin, can be unsafe near mucous membranes, and requires considerable operator skill and proper setup, possibly including an assistant. At higher speeds, the vibratory distraction from our tool swamps out other sensations and, in my experience, is more effective than even spray and stretch.

UNDERSTANDING THE MUSCLE LIBERATOR

So-called massage guns have become a popular consumer item; vendors and articles tout running such tools all over the body to treat muscle soreness. Therapists already using this sort of tool tend to think of it as pounding adhesions and scar tissue out of existence using broad heads and a lot of force. And in general, these devices are used primarily as an automated way to "rub where it hurts."

For instance, if someone with sciatica or "IT band syndrome" uses the tool on the side of their leg, they will likely feel some relief, but it won't last any longer than foam rolling over and over, day in and day out. Unless they understand the origins of sciatic pain, the functional relationships, and satellite referral patterns, they will essentially be treating a symptom rather than the cause, and it will return.

When people see a picture of me working, they're immediately drawn to the tool, as if that is my secret. They want to know where they can buy the tool, a shiny new gadget that can fix their pain. However, we do not sell the tool apart from our training programs because what I care about is changing the way that pain is understood and treated, not selling a piece of hardware that would be ineffective without training, thereby lowering expectations for the success of our approach. The best tool or technique is doomed to mediocrity or outright failure if you don't actually know where the pain comes from and attempt to chase the pain.

One comment I occasionally hear from massage therapists is that tools can't replace hands for massage. I think there's truth to that, but while CTB can be incorporated into a massage practice, Coaching the Body is not massage, nor are we trying to replace human touch. We designed the Muscle Liberator specifically as an accelerator for trigger point therapy, which is quite different. Human hands cannot possibly do what the tool does in terms of vibrating a taut fiber accurately thousands of times per minute or achieve the associated benefits in taut fiber release and neurological distraction. Used in this way, the tool cuts treatment time dramatically and offers results that cannot easily be attained with bodywork alone.

Another misunderstanding I see often is that percussion mechanically "breaks up adhesions," is a replacement for the therapist's body, and that significant force is required. This worldview goes hand in hand with the idea that pain comes from some manner of injury, scar tissue, adhesions, and the like. This viewpoint is simply not accurate. As I mentioned in Chapter 5, taut fibers are contractures in muscle fibers, not scar tissue or fascial hardening. Those things can occur, but the speed with which we can eliminate the vast majority of these hard tissues belies the idea that they are fascial in nature.

We don't use the Muscle Liberator with heavy pressure. This not only wouldn't be helpful but would also, in many cases, hinder the ability of the body to accept the vibratory sensation because it's too intense. Our tool is successful even in highly sensitive areas, such as the neck, because we treat it as a kind of floating vibration rather than something that pounds scar tissue out of existence.

The Muscle Liberator was designed to be an extension of the CTB philosophy. We also manufacture versions of our custom-designed heads that fit the HyperVolt and similar tools. Whatever tool you use, it needs to be applied at the source, not where the pain is felt, or you're wasting your time. The other side of that equation is that if your analysis is good, you can use a variety of tools and techniques to treat each muscle, and you will see substantial benefit. Clearly, the best combination is to have a correct analysis and use an effective, optimal set of techniques for each muscle.

Electronic Point Stimulation

Electroacupuncture was initially developed as an adjunct to needling, and fine electrodes could be clipped to needles to enhance treatment.[41] Companies also began developing single-channel compact units that could provide a pulse via a small probe without

---

41 The electroacupuncture units are generally multichannel square wave pulse generators.

piercing the skin. Some vendors mentioned treating trigger points with these units, but nothing in any detail was published.

While I was a faculty member in the Oriental Body Therapies program at Pacific College of Oriental Medicine many years ago, I was initially fascinated by certain areas of convergence between trigger point therapy and acupuncture. I began experimenting with various electronic point stimulators (EPS) that were developed and used in acupuncture.

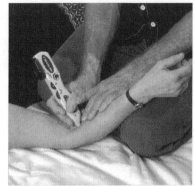

Over the years, I worked with several devices and eventually settled on the Pointer Excel II, which could be held like a pen in one hand. EPS devices work by generating a square wave pulse with controllable intensity and frequency. It contacts the skin via a small ball-shaped tip, making it possible to treat

Fig. 11-3. Using the Pointer Excel II on the brachioradialis in the forearm.

points with precision and accuracy. The body conducts electricity, so if you treat in the region of a motor point, you will often be able to stimulate a series of mini contractions in the target muscle, a phenomenon that I have found to be very clinically effective in treating trigger points, particularly on more superficial muscles with finer fibers, such as muscles of the neck and forearm. I'll go into more detail later in this chapter.

When we use EPS in the vicinity of the motor endplate for a given fiber (generally where trigger points develop), it can pulse the muscle, causing a momentary contraction and release. The therapist must touch the skin while using the EPS, forming a loop in which current flows through the tip and is conducted through the body of the client to the point of touch, where it enters the therapist's body and returns to the device via a metal plate that contacts the therapist's skin. When the specific fibers controlled by the motor point are triggered, they will cause the joint action of that part of the muscle.

For example, when we treat the levator scapulae in its motor endplate zone, the scapula will repeatedly elevate. Essentially, each contraction is like a miniature contract/relax cycle. When this happens, the taut fibers quickly begin to release. There is also a strong analgesic effect, and trigger points that have become very sensitive to touch rapidly lose their sensitivity.

Having used the EPS for over fifteen years in clinical practice, it has become an indispensable tool and my modality of choice for certain muscles. Some muscles, such as levator scapulae, can be difficult to treat with bodywork alone. Tender trigger points in the neck muscles can be hard for patients to tolerate and bring on the protective startle response, which can make things worse. Once the patient gets used to the mild electrical sensation and the pulsing, the EPS quickly calms the muscle. Taut fibers can change in a single treatment cycle without a lot of tender palpation. The EPS tends to work best in smaller, more superficial muscles like the levator because the electric potential is easily carried into the muscle fibers and individual fibers are easy to discriminate.

USING THE EPS

Our treatment cycle with EPS consists of initial palpation to determine taut fibers, treatment of several points, holding twenty to thirty seconds per point, followed by contract/relax. This can produce rapid change. We tend to use EPS extensively in the head and neck, forearm and hand,

Fig. 11-4. EPS example video QR code.

lower leg and foot, shoulder, and certain other relatively superficial muscles with finer fibers, such as vastus medialis. It's also very useful in the abdominal wall, intercostals, and pectoralis major and minor.

For example, when we use EPS on the pectoralis minor, we shorten the pectoralis major and slide the tip under the lateral border of the axilla to contact pectoralis minor fibers directly through the skin. This is incredibly effective and can replace fifteen or twenty minutes of painful bodywork on a shortened pectoralis minor with treatment that lasts a few minutes and leaves the muscle soft and the shoulder less protracted.

It's important to know muscle fiber direction and extent when using the EPS. Some muscles have complex fiber arrangements with oblique or multipennate fibers. For a longitudinal type of muscle, the muscle's geographic centerline is very similar to the fiber centerlines. For a bipennate arrangement such as in the rectus femoris, there are angled fibers on each side, so the physiological centerline is really two lines that converge.

If we discover a taut fiber when palpating across the fiber direction, we begin the EPS treatment with the tip near that centerline. We make contact with the tip, press the treatment button, and then move the tip slightly to explore where we get the most vivid motor effects. We generally use a pulse frequency of four to eight cycles per second, each pulse creating a contraction and release. The combination of electrical activity at the neuromuscular junction and the mechanical contract and release cycle is extremely effective at clearing trigger points.

Although we tend to use it primarily on superficial fibers, the EPS signal can penetrate tissues and influence deep muscles. It is less convenient for large, bulky muscles like the glutes and quadriceps (although it does work well with the small fibers of the oblique belly of vastus medialis). We detail the muscles for which EPS is most appropriate in our Muscle Manual and protocols. For many muscles, both the Muscle Liberator and EPS are useful options.

"I first got into yoga when I was in my early thirties and very active playing competitive soccer and basketball. Though I was in good shape from working out regularly, running, and playing sports, I was still prone to experiencing crippling bouts of low back pain from no injury or cause that I could discern. Every six to twelve months, I would wake up and not be able to move without intense back pain. When this happened, I would very slowly roll off the bed onto my hands and knees and crawl. I would eventually make it to standing erect and then walking, but each step held the possibility of stabbing pain and low back 'spasm' until everything calmed down over a few days. If things didn't get better, I would go to a chiropractor for a couple weeks, and the drop table adjustments would help get me to normal again.

"The chiropractor suggested that yoga could help my back, so I started going to classes and trying different styles, and it did help. I got into the habit of doing four to five Bikram classes per week, a substantial time commitment. I found as long as I continued this, my back felt great, and I had no pain episodes, but if I stopped, my back would start to 'act up.' This sent me on a mission of exploring physical yoga as well as the whole yoga spiritual science in an effort to better understand my body, mind, and pain.

"I eventually did a yoga training at the Temple of Kriya Yoga in Chicago and became a certified teacher and started teaching. I learned a lot in those nine months of training, and I read every anatomy book on yoga I could find and even studied physical therapy textbooks. But I still had a frustrating lack of understanding of the sources of my own back pain. And most students coming to my classes were there to address their own specific pain issues, which I could sympathize with but couldn't significantly understand or help with, except in the most general way. It was all a big guessing game, and I don't like guessing.

"I kept searching for answers and asking everyone I knew where I could learn anatomy. I took yoga anatomy workshops and explored massage and physical therapy schools. Fortuitously, a yoga teacher friend recommended Chuck Duff, who taught Clinical Thai Bodywork (which eventually became Coaching the Body). I took his anatomy class and was blown away. This was the knowledge I had been searching for. He understood the true sources of pain and movement dysfunction and proved it every time he worked with a client or student—on the spot—making huge reductions in pain and increasing mobility in minutes. I needed to know everything he did, so I started studying and apprenticing with him and eventually became a CTB teacher and helped evolve the system and teaching.

"Because of my athletic past, daily yoga practice, and personal pain history, I have always had a particular interest in applying the CTB knowledge to athletic training, yoga, self-care, and rehabilitation. I am pain-free now, except for the rare occasion I overload my low back/hip muscles by slipping on an icy mountain trail, for example. If I do get a pain issue, I can quickly resolve it using CTB self-care and CTB-informed yoga.

"The CTB knowledge revolutionized my yoga practice and yoga teaching. When I feel a pain sensation in an asana, instead of assuming there is a local problem or injury, I can visualize what muscles are shortening/lengthening and eccentrically stabilizing and cross reference that in my mind with the pain referral patterns and figure out the muscle sources of the pain sensation. If there is a movement limitation from pain, I can address it and move the barrier within seconds by contracting the source muscle for five to seven seconds while holding a breath, then releasing the breath, relaxing the muscle, and lengthening it passively or actively (contract/relax stretch). I can also add vibration on the stretch or do some feedback compression if needed for further effect.

"I can do the same thing with students in a yoga class, change their experience, and move their barrier on the spot with manual feedback compression on the limiting muscle and/or verbal instruction, instead of just offering them a bailout (not therapeutic). The most rewarding thing to me is showing someone how they can treat their own pain issues with yoga and/or other self-care techniques. That comes from understanding pain and anatomy through CTB.

"I have applied the CTB knowledge to my clients' self-care, rehabilitation, and athletic training as well as my own with great success.
My personal daily practice is designed as a diagnostic 'flight check'
as well as a balancing and strengthening maintenance program. I am
a very hyper-mobile person and need balanced muscular strength
to stabilize my joints to keep me pain-free. Because of the CTB
knowledge, I know the weak links in my kinetic chain and how to
strengthen them. If I encounter an issue during a movement, I have a
myriad of ways to address it with a CTB self-care technique or asana/
exercise variation that works therapeutically with the limitation and
with very quick results."

—Doug Ringwald, CTB master practitioner and instructor and
NASM Corrective Exercise Specialist

CHAPTER 12

Self-Treatment with CTB

While we're working steadily to train more practitioners in our revolutionary approach, it can still be hard to find therapists who are familiar with our system and adequately trained to achieve consistent results. If you're unable to find a CTB-trained therapist, you can apply the principles of CTB quite well to self-care. As is the case with our bodywork approach, we have developed effective self-care techniques.

Understanding where issues originate from is the key to solving them. With a willingness to learn and be methodical, you can accomplish a lot on your own. We've developed self-care courses for shoulder pain and sciatica, and people get great results with them.

This chapter highlights some techniques that you can use on yourself while applying the principles of CTB. Much of the material in this chapter is excerpted from our online courses, Treat Your Own Shoulder Pain and Treat Your Own Sciatica & Hip Pain. I won't go into specific strategies for self-care, but for more information on our self-care resources, scan the QR code in Figure 12-1.

Fig. 12-1. Self-care example video QR code.

When using CTB for self-care, we apply the same basic treatment cycle, but instead of relying on a therapist to move your joints, you'll have to actively move your own. We also apply contract/

relax, which works quite well and we rely on heavily throughout the treatment. In general, we work muscles into short, through range, and then do contract/relax to stretch.

You can use a variety of tools to provide compression. Tiger Tail balls are excellent, and we distribute them with our self-care courses. Vibration is still one of the most effective techniques; at CTBI, we all reach first for the Muscle Liberator when working on our own bodies. While compression with a ball or cane can feel tender, the vibration can minimize tenderness, and the neurological distraction is just as important for yourself as it is when working on someone else's body.

Best Strategies for Self-Treatment Success

Most approaches to bodywork and self-care have the primary strategy of compressing the areas where pain is felt and moving the point of compression around but not the muscle. A prime example of this is using a foam roller on the outside of the thigh, as discussed in Chapter 6. They move the foam roller repeatedly across areas where they experience muscle pain. This approach fails to apply some key principles for long-term pain relief. As you learn to apply CTB principles and techniques to your own body, remember these guidelines for the best results:

1. Understand where the pain is generated. Most importantly, know not to apply compression in the wrong place. "Rubbing it where it hurts" is not useful; as we learned earlier, pain is often caused by a trigger point somewhere else in the body. When someone experiences pain that they associate with their IT band, it has nothing to do with the IT band and most likely not even the muscle that lies underneath it (vastus lateralis). For each common pain pattern in our self-care

protocols, we guide you through the sequence of muscles that could be relevant in terms of both satellite referral and functional relationships.

2. Compression with movement is better than passive rolling. Moving the roller but not the muscle you're compressing is another unhelpful strategy. The whole idea of "rolling" is somewhat flawed. Rolling over tender areas means that you're not spending much time actually compressing the trigger points, and you're also not retraining the muscle to be able to change length. It's a far better approach to find the right area, then hold compression on it while you move the joint associated with the muscle, which changes the length of the muscle.

3. Find the hard fibers. The most efficient way to find trigger points is to look for hard fibers—areas of muscle that feel ropy—and then follow along the length of the fiber until you find a tender area (normally near the attachments of that particular hard fiber). Sometimes it's a good idea to explore a little with your fingertips first, and then apply a compression technique suited for that area.

4. Pure compression isn't nearly as effective as vibration. As mentioned earlier, a vibration tool distracts the nervous system, making the body less likely to generate the pain that you normally feel. This allows more thorough treatment with less pain, meaning the body will permit the muscles to release and move more quickly and easily.

About Pain and Tenderness during Treatment

When you locate a trigger point area in your muscles, it will most likely feel tender where you compress it. It might also cause referral—that is, pain or other sensations elsewhere in your body. For example, the infraspinatus muscle in the back of the shoulder causes pain in the front of the shoulder when you press or stretch it. Even so, it's important to remember that self-care is not self-torture. There is no need to suffer through extreme pain as you treat your own muscles. In fact, pain is counterproductive because your nervous system will ultimately go into self-protective mode instead of opening up.

While it's normal to feel tenderness and often referral during self-treatment, remember to keep it at a tolerable level. We use a 1–10 pain scale in our bodywork. One means that you hardly feel anything, while 10 would mean horrific pain. In between—5 or 6—is still tolerable, but approaching a point at which your body starts to experience tension and stress. When compressing tender points, you should keep pain to a tolerable 3 or 4 on a scale of 10. If your face is scrunching up and you're tightening your muscles, it's too much. Compression doesn't need to go on for a long time; it's far better to do a few minutes with movement and intersperse your compression work with contract/relax.

Some joints are far more sensitive than others and are more likely to lock down and go into a protective mode. For example, the shoulder is particularly vulnerable to adaptive locking down of muscle fibers, due to its natural mobility and lack of hard structure, resulting in extreme pain and loss of pain-free movement. Often the descriptive term "frozen shoulder" is simply the end game of this process, in which the body has gone through a progressive adaptation in the muscles that stabilize the scapula and arm. When working on yourself, you should stay on the gentle side and take care not to set yourself back by triggering the body's protective response.

Another advantage provided by vibration tools is that they can provide compression with less pain. If you're not using a vibration tool, just decrease your pressure until you are at a 3 or 4 level. Focus on moving the muscle and holding compression rather than rolling over tender areas and constantly causing yourself a lot of pain.

Often it is beneficial to press on any areas where you feel pain away from the site of compression. We call this feedback, which we do in therapy quite often. The pressure will distract the nervous system and allow you to move through more range without pain.

We've developed appropriate techniques for each muscle, but there is far too much material to cover here. You can view video examples of self-treatment by scanning the QR code in this section, or visiting coachingthebody.com/selfcare/.

Movement and Stretching

Most people misunderstand the effects of stretching and how to use stretch when caring for their own muscles. Someone with an active stretching practice—whose muscles are conditioned to change length on a regular basis—can tolerate more stretching earlier with fewer negative effects than someone who doesn't. But if the muscles haven't been moving a lot (because of pain or immobility), simple stretching often irritates muscles with trigger points. When you stretch a muscle with trigger points, it's likely that you will cause the muscle's pain referral pattern to occur, and you might feel some pain in the muscle itself. As we know, once the body experiences pain, it tends to create protective engagement, which will make it much harder to get a "productive" stretch that allows the fibers to release. It's important to treat the tender areas in the muscle first with compression or vibration, then use a therapeutic type of stretching called contract/relax.

Contract/relax uses a basic physiological principle to great advantage. Just after you make a muscle work by engaging it, that muscle is much more likely to stretch effectively. This is a "hack" that was initially discovered by osteopaths and finds use in sports medicine and some movement disciplines.

The first phase is making the muscle work, meaning that you engage it with a mild effort—10 to 20 percent of full contraction—against some resistance. Hold the engagement for five or more seconds while you hold an inhale. The second phase makes the muscle lengthen; as you let out the breath, you stretch the muscle. In CTB work, we use vibration during the stretch phase to distract the nervous system and produce a more effective stretch with less discomfort.

Self-Treatment Protocols

At CTBI, we've developed detailed self-treatment protocols for the most common pain conditions in the upper and lower body. We offer online self-care courses as part of our digital course library, either alone or bundled with the purchase of vibration tools and compression balls. Please visit coachingthebody.com/selfcare/ for details.

> "Lisa came to the CTB clinic with top right shoulder pain, stiff neck, and pain when turning her head to the right. She used to enjoy attending yoga classes, but always struggled with asanas that challenged the shoulder muscles. Arm balances were out of the question. She also avoided doing downward facing dog and chaturanga because they would light up her shoulder/neck pain. She would sit those poses out in classes and replace them with ones that didn't use arm/shoulders.
>
> "She had head and shoulder forward positioning due to foot hyperpronation, which we addressed with corrective insoles. She also had a leg length discrepancy, the compensation from which kept her right shoulder higher than the left. This partly explained why she had pain on the right shoulder and pain on turning her head to the right

but not the left. The levator scapula muscle stabilizes the neck and shoulder and commonly produces pain referral to the crook of the neck when it is shortened by turning the head to the same side. She was also right hand dominant, and worked at a computer without proper elbow support, which requires the scapular elevators to work hard. I discussed a different workstation arrangement with her.

"I used the CTB shoulder protocol to treat the neck and scapular stabilizers. The top of the shoulder pain on the right side had significant contribution from the scapular stabilizers (serratus anterior and trapezius) which is often the case. These muscles had significant trigger points that stabilized her shoulder forward positioning. The trigger points in her serratus anterior and trapezius also explained why downward facing dog and other asanas that challenged her scapular stabilizers caused neck and shoulder pain. These muscles were functionally weak from the trigger points and needed to be rehabilitated. After some bodywork sessions along with CTB self-care for the scapular stabilizers, the active pain was gone and it was time to progress to incremental strengthening.

"We used the Mighty Body Band to do strengthening sets for the scapular stabilizers as well as end every set with a contract/relax stretch for the muscles she just worked. This helped reduce the possibility of muscular overload, which would be a set back and cause active pain. When she did get pain, we stopped and did bodywork to relieve it right away. She moved on to doing downward facing dog using the MBB hip belt to manage how much work the shoulders had to do in the pose. She was then able to progress to more upper body challenging yoga work as well as weight lifting on her own."

—Doug Ringwald, CTB master practitioner and instructor and NASM Corrective Exercise Specialist

CHAPTER 13

Perpetuating Factors: Understanding the Inputs

Although the methods I've described in the previous chapters have proven very effective at eliminating pain in most conditions we see, the pain is likely to return if we don't understand what caused it in the first place. Problematic trigger points do not arise randomly; they're often a response to stresses, chronic or acute, that affect the muscular system.

When working with a client, they must complete a thorough intake form so that we can do some detective work on what adaptations the body has taken. The intake form should ask questions about their lifestyle, medical history, and more, such as:

- Type of work they do, including any mechanical and/or emotional stresses

- Hobbies, sports, and exercise

- Sleep habits and position

- Home/family environment and stresses

- Medications

- Food, nutrition, and hydration

- Past pain, injuries, surgeries, and diagnoses

- Eyewear and/or vision issues

Once we know more about the client, we can begin to paint a picture that allows us to assess the stress factors that their body and nervous system face. You might find it useful to complete an intake form for yourself if you're using the self-care techniques mentioned in the previous chapter.

I've found that there are several key perpetuating factors that can cause recurring and potentially persistent pain in the body: leg length discrepancy, hemipelvis discrepancy, hyperpronation in the feet, and breathing dysfunction. In this chapter, I'll explain each of these factors, as well as how to mitigate the chronic pain that they might cause.

Leg Length Discrepancy

In the twenty years I've spent developing CTB, I've observed an extremely high correlation between unilateral pain in the lower body and leg length discrepancy (LLD), starting with myself. This pain is often related to dysfunction in the QL, one of several muscles extremely sensitive to lateral asymmetry. The QL ties the torso and spine to the hips, and it can develop trigger points if it rests at a different length than its partner on the opposite side.[42] LLD is common, and yet it is often overlooked and misunderstood.

---

42 The original Travell and Simons *Volume 2* (1992) has an extensive discussion of lower limb length inequality in relation to the quadratus lumborum. See page 45.

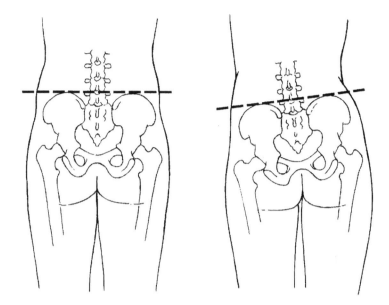

Fig. 13-1. Sacral tilt as a result of effective leg length discrepancy.

Most people have a hard time believing that even a difference of a quarter of an inch could disturb their muscles so thoroughly that they end up with severe sciatic pain. In addition, many people have gone to other practitioners who diagnose them with some other condition or treat them with methods that don't bring reliable relief. For example, a client might already have orthotic inserts in their shoes, but their pain hasn't subsided. Others (including myself) might have been told that their asymmetry is a reflection of a spinal issue, and they need to return to have their spine adjusted once or twice a week for basically the rest of their lives.

My Own Leg Length Discrepancy

I use my own body as the proving ground for many of my ideas. I had the curse/opportunity of severe pain as a young man, which motivated me to investigate these ideas and gave me a terrific laboratory to try things out. For many years when I was younger, I would experience painful spasms in my low back, with pain sometimes wrapping around to the front and radiating down my leg. I visited my chiropractor twice a week. He would measure my leg length as I lay prone on the table, tap my L3-4 vertebrae (in the mid-back) back into alignment, and said that his adjustments corrected the difference. His adjustments reduced the recurrent pain episodes but didn't eliminate them. He had to do the same adjustment every time, so he wasn't correcting anything, just maintaining a temporary alignment that would inevitably return to an imbalanced state.

Evaluating Leg Length Discrepancy

Actual bony lower limb length inequality of over 5mm has been observed in approximately 50 percent of various populations,[43] making it, and the unilateral pain it can cause, quite common. Unfortunately, evaluation of lower limb length is seriously misunderstood. I find that most clients who have been evaluated for leg length have been evaluated while lying on a table, like I was when I was younger. This approach doesn't make sense.

When the client isn't bearing weight on their feet, you include the effect of the muscles that control pelvic lateral tilt (primarily the QL), unfettered by joint stacking and gravity. If one QL has trigger points and shortening due to taut fibers, it will pull the hip up closer to the ribs and possibly even make that leg appear shorter on the table. The QL on the long side is most likely to develop

43 Travell and Simons, *Myofascial Pain and Dysfunction: The Trigger Point Manual Vol. 2., The Lower Extremities*, 56–58.

trigger points and become adaptively shortened, and when someone is lying on a table, this QL dysfunction can actually cause the long leg to appear shorter.

Fig. 13-2.
Evaluating LLD
QR code.

When someone who has LLD stands and is weight-bearing, the sacrum will end up tilted to one side, causing it to be imbalanced during walking. While standing, the longer leg will raise the hip and cause the QL on that side to rest at a shorter length than the other, making it somewhat lax. Laxity on one side is inherently unstable, and, as you now know, the body abhors instability. The fibers of the shortened QL often develop trigger points as a means of adaptive shortening, bringing tone back to the shortened fibers. Often, symptoms are worse on the long side with the shortened QL, but it all depends upon how the client's body adapts to their specific lateral asymmetry. In any case, both QLs will see some level of disturbance.

In our assessment, which is done standing and weight-bearing, we measure the effective leg length—the sum total of bony differences, joint play and alignment, hyperpronation, and more—not the actual anatomical lengths of the bones. We aren't doing any radiology; we're examining the effective height at the top of the iliac crest, which summarizes the sizes of the femur, the lower leg, ankle, and foot, as well as joint play, any left to right differences in hyperpronation, and potential adaptive pelvic nutation. What's important is whether the sacrum is tilted or not and whether forces during gait are uneven.

We have the client stand with their feet close together in front of a level line that we could use as a visual reference near their waist level. We place our hands with straight fingers held out like a blade above the top of the iliac crest, ensuring that we are on top of the pelvis and not pressing into it from the side. By comparing our hands to the level sightline, we can tell if there is a difference and roughly how much it might be. We then use boards of one-eighth of an inch to build up a correction and place it under one side and then the other. When the boards are placed under the side that appears short, the goal is to bring the tops of the iliac crest as even as possible.

We ask the client for a subjective report with the correction on each side to verify our findings. Often the client will initially report that it is uncomfortably different than they are used to on the side that needs correction. We then move the correction to the other side and come back to compare. Once the client experiences the long side being pushed up even farther, they will report that the corrected side feels good. There are many subtleties to this procedure; please scan the QR code in Figure 13-2 and see our video example for more detail.

SCOLIOSIS

Many cases of scoliosis can be traced to the effects of lateral asymmetry tilting the base of the spine. If the sacrum is tilted, the upper body musculature will compensate, sometimes in unpredictable ways. A relatively small tilt can trigger larger regional curvatures, with hypertonic muscles alternating to maintain balance, culminating in the cervical spine, which may exhibit a curve as well. The body will usually attempt to level the eyes, but the shoulders and the cervical (neck), thoracic, and lumbar spine may all exhibit curvatures. For this reason, LLD can influence any pain region in the body, from sciatic pain to low back, mid back, shoulder, and head/neck pain.

SCIATICA AND LEG LENGTH DISCREPANCY

The seemingly unrelated collection of complaints called "sciatica" confuses most practitioners. Because sciatic pain patterns often roughly resemble nerve patterns, most people assume that an impinged or entrapped nerve is responsible, so they blame the sciatic nerve, primarily because of its name. In truth, the name "sciatic" came via Latin from the Greek "ischiadikos," which means "subject to trouble in the hips or loins." The name of the nerve and the symptom both derive from this root, but no causal connection is implied. Travell was careful to point out that the term sciatica is not a diagnosis but simply a common pain pattern connoting radiation down the leg.[44] In actuality, nothing about the name sciatica implies or reveals the true source of the pain; it's just a symptom.

Sciatic pain can be crippling. We have seen hundreds of severe cases of sciatica, and we get reliably excellent results with our bodywork approach, generally with significant relief in the first session. Many have been to multiple practitioners without relief. Based on these experiences, I'm confident in the process of analysis described here, following the intersection of function and satellite referral. The influence of lateral asymmetry on upper body issues can be dramatic as well. Ultimately, even with the best bodywork, if nothing changes in perpetuating factors, nothing changes with the pain. Analyzing and correcting perpetuating factors is the key to keeping the pain from returning.

In order to fully appreciate the far-reaching effects of the body's adaptations to lateral asymmetry, we have to consider the satellite referral patterns involved. In the lower body, QL refers into the gluteal muscles, particularly the gluteus medius and minimus. The gluteus minimus is known in trigger point therapy as the "sciatica

---

44 Travell and Simons, *Myofascial Pain and Dysfunction: The Trigger Point Manual; Vol. 2., The Lower Extremities*, 173.

muscle." The gluteus medius is the most common source of low back pain, and its referral pattern goes directly over the QL.

In a client with LLD, the gluteus minimus and medius will be subject to both functional and satellite influences. Trigger points in one or both QLs will cause satellite referral into the corresponding glutes and TFL. If bombarded by satellite referral, the gluteus minimus can initiate the radiating leg pain pattern that is commonly identified as sciatica. The QL also stabilizes the lumbar spine and neurologically is in a complex relationship with the deep erector spinae, such as multifidi, which provide local segmental stabilization. The composite referral patterns of the QL, gluteus medius and minimus, and TFL amount to a full-blown and often crippling sciatic pain pattern: low back, gluteal, hip, abdominal, and thigh pain. Due to the phenomenon of joint coupling, any side bending in the lumbar spine is accompanied by a rotational component.[45]

If one hip is higher and the sacrum tilts due to LLD, there will be three-dimensional effects on the segments and deep stabilizers of the lumbar spine beyond simple lateral tilting. If a vertebral segment rotates, it may then subtly or not so subtly compress a nerve, and some of the nerves that emerge from the spine adjacent to the QL fibers actually innervate the QL. When nerves are compressed, they tend to cause dysfunction and produce trigger points in the muscles they innervate. In these cases, the QL may receive additional stress from the addition of neurological involvement to the basic problems of asymmetric resting length produced by LLD.

The gluteal muscles can be in for a double dose of disturbance from LLD. The glutes are key stabilizers of the leg during the weight-bearing phase of gait. Lateral asymmetry causes subtle differences between the left and right abductors of the hip during gait, as they hold the pelvis up when weight-bearing and assist in

45 Carol A. Oatis, *Kinesiology: The Mechanics and Pathomechanics of Human Movement*, 3rd ed. (Philadelphia: Wolters Kluwer, 2017), 1891–1893.

swinging the leg through after the other leg plants. (Hyperpronation, which we will cover in a later section, also demands additional stabilization from the glutes.) These functional stressors can set the glutes up for dysfunction and promote the development of taut fibers without any other factors being involved. Satellite referral from the QL then becomes an additional stress. I believe that this combination of functional stressors and satellite referral makes these muscles highly vulnerable and is why they are so impactful in lower body pain.

When the gluteal fibers become compromised with trigger points, they can become functionally weak. This means that during gait, the gluteal abduction fibers cannot fulfill their role of hip leveling and supporting swing-through of the leg as effectively. In these cases, the TFL tries to assist and substitute for compromised glutes, which can overload it and perpetuate dysfunction. Because the TFL is a hybrid muscle (abduction and hip flexion), it can't take on a substantial load of hip stabilization. The QL can also assist, somewhat ineffectively, by substituting hip hiking for gluteal abduction. This phenomenon—in which secondary muscles take over when the primary agonist can't do its job—is a well-known adaptation that can establish trigger points due to overload in some key areas of the body.

This sensitive configuration of muscular stabilizers in the lumbar spine amplifies the effects of LLD. All of these factors can cause the pain that is commonly diagnosed as sciatica. Personally, I suffered transient, severe episodes of deep lumbar pain accompanied by sciatic pain for many years until I became aware of how to assess and correct for LLD.

CORRECTING LEG LENGTH DISCREPANCY

The goal of correction is to bring the sacrum to a nominally level position, and the easiest way to do so is with a heel lift or full footbed lift in the client's shoe. Even though the client won't be in the correction 100 percent of the time, if they prioritize the shoes that they wear and walk in the most, the lift will reduce the asymmetric load on the lumbar muscles and glutes and could be enough to keep them below the threshold of active pain. Adding lifts to my own shoes made a huge difference for me, to the point that I no longer have recurring low back pain. I've found that tweaks of as little as an eighth of an inch can make a significant difference.

If I see someone for the first time presenting with some aspect of a unilateral sciatic pattern, I always do the lateral asymmetry assessments. Often, I do bodywork first and then assess their leg length. That removes any contribution of hypertonic muscles from the equation, although weight-bearing assessment minimizes any muscular component of the asymmetry. In addition, it's important to reassess LLD on a regular basis. While bony lengths don't change, soft tissue elements can. It is best to reassess the client on their corrections in their preferred shoes.

Hemipelvis Discrepancy

The bones of the pelvis can also exhibit developmental asymmetry. The hemipelvis consists of the bones of the pelvis on one side, and if it develops asymmetrically, the distance from the sit bone to the top of the sacrum will be different on the two sides. For individuals who sit on relatively firm, level surfaces for several hours, this imbalance causes a tilted sacrum; softer surfaces tend to absorb the pressure and mask the difference.

Hemipelvis discrepancy can cause similar pain as leg length discrepancy. Since the QL resting length will be different on the two sides, one or both QL muscles could develop trigger points and refer pain into the glutes, initiating the satellite referral-based sciatic pattern discussed above. However, unlike LLD, hemipelvis discrepancy causes more pain in the upper body: in the torso, shoulder, head, and neck—areas also related to spinal and shoulder asymmetries.

Correction in these cases is less formal than with LLD because soft seat cushions are far more forgiving than hard floors. A folded towel or cloth under the sit bone on the smaller side can be sufficient when the client is working or driving.

Hyperpronation

The feet and ankles establish our contact with the ground, so variations in foot and ankle anatomy can set up severe and persistent patterns of dysfunction in the body. Travell and Simons focused on the Morton foot structure as a source of instability rather than hyperpronation. However, in practice, we have found hyperpronation to be the more common source of pain. That said, there is significant overlap between Morton's foot and hyperpronation.

MORTON'S FOOT STRUCTURE

Morton's foot structure describes an anatomical variation in which the second metatarsal is longer than the first and third, which can create biomechanical instability. This condition is sometimes called "Morton's toe" because the long second metatarsal can cause the second toe to be longer than the first. While the ancient Greeks found this structure aesthetically pleasing, it can cause chronic pain in the body.

Normally, the foot should operate as a tripod, with pressure behind the big toe and two smallest toes (the distal ends of the first and fifth metatarsals) and on the heel. As the heel lifts during gait and weight transfers into the forefoot, a long second metatarsal adds an extra vertex near the center of the ball of the foot, causing weight to focus on the head of the second metatarsal rather than the first and fifth. Because the second metatarsal is making contact with the ground, the foot wobbles side to side and the muscles in the foot, leg, and hip must engage to stabilize the foot. Someone with Morton's foot may overuse the toe flexors while attempting to stabilize, along with the long flexors, extensors, and other muscles of the lower leg. More importantly, the gluteal and adductor muscles of the hip may come into play, setting up sciatic, knee, and groin pain.

HYPERPRONATION: HYPERMOBILITY OF THE ANKLE

Hyperpronation is different from Morton's foot structure, but it is very closely related and seems to be extremely common in the US. It may have to do with early development and children wearing shoes on hard surfaces early in life, but that is only speculation. Whatever its origin, the issue is so common that we assess virtually every client. I have found proper correction using our insole system to effectively reduce ongoing pain. I wear the insoles in all of my shoes and can feel it immediately if I don't. Correcting my hyperpronation and effective LLD (along with an exercise protocol to maintain deep lumbar stability) has kept me away from the severe, recurring pain that plagued me when I was younger.

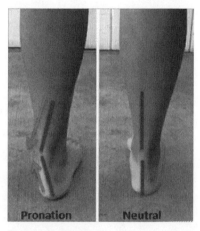

Fig. 13-3. Hyperpronation at the ankle. Credit: Ducky2315, CC BY-SA 3.0, via Wikimedia Commons.

Pronation is a necessary movement of the ankle that provides for smooth weight transfer during gait. As we shift weight into the foot, the foot everts, meaning that the arch drops a bit and the entire foot tilts medially and also turns away from the center line—or abducts. It is important to have sufficient mobility in the ligaments of the foot and ankle to support this motion. However, if the ligaments do not properly constrain movement, various muscles will be recruited to provide stability, ranging from short intrinsic muscles in the foot to longer movers of the ankle to powerful remote muscles, including the TFL, glutes, and adductors.

Standing at rest, a hyperpronator may appear to have flat arches. However, a true collapsed arch is a different and much more unusual situation. A severely hyperpronated foot appears to have no arch, but if the eversion of the foot is corrected, the arch will return. From behind, the heel and Achilles tendon can often be seen to curve inward as the foot everts.

Most individuals will unconsciously employ muscle engagement to keep the arch from collapsing in, which becomes a muscular habit of over-engagement. When you assess a patient who does this, they are probably not even aware that it's happening. If you can really get them to relax, they will let their ankles hyperpronate, and it will feel so unpleasant to them that they will revert to engagement.

This chronic over-engagement has consequences. We've discussed how effective LLD can cause dysfunction in the QL and gluteal muscles, which have a cross-referral relationship with each other. Hyperpronation can also add stress to the glutes as the individual uses the abduction power of the glutes to prevent the arch from dropping medially and the knee from moving into valgus (commonly referred to as "knock knees").

While a majority of hyperpronators tend to manage the hyperpronation via muscular engagement, which causes pain and dysfunction in the lower body, others might suffer pain in the upper body as a result of postural collapse. The inward collapse at the ankles sets up a chain of joint actions causing postural changes, including anterior pelvic tilt, excess lordosis, and thoracic kyphosis, culminating in protracted shoulders and forward head. As the torso and head come forward, the spinal erectors and neck muscles must work harder to restrain the collapse.

THE PERILS OF STRENGTHENING AS A SOLE STRATEGY

In my experience, therapists tend to assume that strengthening a particular muscle that appears weak will restore its functional balance and relieve pain. A great deal is written about strengthening the glutes to prevent valgus knee. However, hyperpronation can cause valgus knee, so this guidance misses the vital point that if someone's ankle is unstable and has a tendency to collapse inward, they will either let it happen (causing the knees to move into a valgus position) or engage their glutes to force stability from above by abducting the entire leg and bringing the weight more to the outside of the foot. Everyday walking can further embed trigger points in the glute fibers, making them functionally weak.

Instructing the person to use exercise bands or complete abduction exercises will further overload compromised fibers. Most people will abandon a strength program if it perpetuates or worsens their severe pain. Many of the patients who come through our doors have been failed by this kind of strengthening regimen, which can worsen their sciatic pain due to the referral of the gluteus minimus, causing the typical pain pattern identified as sciatica. In general, due to their stabilizing role during gait, the glutes tend to get plenty of use in someone who is active. Gluteal weakness is a misguided assessment in most cases as a cause of either valgus knee or sciatica.

Of course, strength is a good thing, but how you get there is critical. Muscles severely compromised by embedded taut fibers will not respond well to immediate strengthening exercises. The muscle must be reconditioned with an effective trigger point therapy first. Then, strength training must be incremental. In CTB, we incorporate our self-care techniques into strengthening so that any overloaded fibers are constantly being rehabilitated. Once the taut fibers are treated, the glutes will immediately exhibit significantly more functional strength.

USING CORRECTIONS

Many people have reservations about using corrections versus developing enough strength for the muscles to handle the overstabilization without overload and trigger points. I very much appreciate this viewpoint because it's consistent with my own passion about becoming independent and not jumping to symptomatic solutions. I support the idea of developing strength. However, in practice, hyperpronation is extremely difficult to treat through strengthening alone and is unlikely to overcome the sheer chronic volume of stress from gait disturbance through thousands of steps per day. To do so requires sophisticated training, with scenarios in which the foot must adapt to irregular and unstable surfaces to train the muscles of the foot and ankle, which must be done incrementally so as not to produce trigger points and set the body back. Even if successful, an individual would have to follow this regimen throughout their entire life.

We have to be realistic about what the typical client is willing and able to do. I have some highly motivated clients who would do anything I ask, but for many, the basic demands of making a living, raising a family, and maintaining a home take priority. In addition, most of us have walked around in shoes on hard surfaces since childhood, which is not a great proprioceptive environment for muscles that evolved to adapt to fluid, irregular surfaces.

Before trying any kind of corrections, we first do rehabilitative bodywork on the glutes/QL/adductor complex. Many people will have a different degree of hyperpronation in their right and left feet, which can contribute to effective leg length differences. For this reason, it is helpful to correct hyperpronation before settling on a leg length correction.

Then we assess and correct hyperpronation with insole supports under the arch, first metatarsal, and in severe cases, potentially the heel. These supports are not a crutch. They allow the glutes to remain strong and do their job without the extra load of stabilizing against hyperpronation. Once the correction has been put in place during an assessment, it isn't unusual for the client to state that they feel much taller and are visibly standing more upright. Additional strength training at that point may be productive. The goal of corrections is to provide sufficient support and proprioceptive feedback so the instinct to hold the ankle rigid and supinate is greatly reduced. Having to hold the foot in supination is one of the most powerful stressors of the gluteal fibers, leading to sciatic pain, hip, low back pain, and more.

I experimented with having clients use off-the-shelf insoles for a few years. Ultimately, we were forced to design our own because the existing products didn't accomplish our goal of calming the muscles of the kinetic chain that respond to instability in the ankle. Most were only suitable for mild hyperpronators, provided too little support in the arch, and lacked options for correction in the first metatarsal or heel. Our Hyperpronation Correction System can provide correction in all of these areas and is easily modified and customized. Scan the QR code in Figure 13-4 or visit

Fig. 13-4. Hyper-pronation and correction video QR code.

https://coachingthebody.com/book-pronation-collapse for more information.

Some clients often come in with custom orthotics, but most of them have had a negative experience with them, finding that they don't help. Orthotics are designed so that the only correction is in the heel and midfoot. The front is either cut off or is a flexible flap, so they don't accommodate first metatarsal correction. I've seen cases in which the head of the first metatarsal was hollowed out because the patient had a painful first joint. In effect, this was dropping the forefoot into pronation and failing to provide proprioceptive feedback on the first joint.[46]

Breathing Dysfunction

Breathing involves expanding the volume of the lungs, creating a vacuum, and allowing air to flow in. The most energy-efficient way of accomplishing this is for the diaphragm to expand the lungs by pulling the inferior membrane, or pleura, down into the abdominal cavity. When we do so, the diaphragm pushes into our internal organs, causing them to expand the belly.

We can also increase lung volume by expanding the ribcage. This action requires much more effort because we must move the ribs. They can expand lung volume by pivoting forward and to

---

46 Some custom orthotics are created by machines that measure the weightbearing characteristics of the client's foot, which has become a significant side business for some practitioners. However, the machine only measures where the client puts weight using their compensatory strategy. The machine might identify some clients as "supinators" because they brace and throw all of their weight to the outside of the foot. The client is actually compensating for hyperpronation, but the machine may decide that their supination requires correction, which is the opposite of what they actually need. The subtalar joint is made to facilitate pronation. So-called supinators are not being made to supinate by their ankle anatomy, barring a severe injury or anatomical aberration. I have seen ankles reconstructed after being badly broken, and in some cases the repair forced them into supination.

the sides at their vertebral joints. This requires muscles higher in the thorax to pull them up, known as ancillary breathing muscles, because supporting inspiration is not their primary function. Any muscle that connects to the ribs below and the spine or shoulder girdle above is capable of assisting with this type of breath, such as the scalenes, pectoralis minor, high trapezius, sternocleidomastoids, intercostals, serratus posterior superior, and serratus anterior.

CHEST BREATHING AND SHOULDER PAIN

When we're exerting ourselves—such as when running—our diaphragm should initiate high-demand breathing. The ancillary breathing muscles in the upper chest and neck assist in later stages. In these cases, we need all possible help to get enough oxygen into our system. Unless you're running a marathon or doing some other long-form aerobic activity, the body should only use the ancillary breathing muscles for a short period of time. We call this action "chest breathing."

Chest breathing seems innocuous and tends to go unnoticed. When patients develop a habit of chest breathing as a dominant strategy, failing to employ the diaphragm to do its job, chest breathing can produce dramatic symptoms by overloading some of the most potent muscles in the body for producing pain. These habits can develop early in life, sometimes as a way of looking good and keeping a flat stomach. The high muscles of the chest and shoulders are smaller than the diaphragm and have other primary functions, which do not include breathing. For this reason, they are easily overloaded.

The scalenes are very vulnerable to overuse through habitual high chest breathing. They are small muscles that connect the cervical column to the first two ribs, which allows them to lift the rib cage from above and participate in expanding the volume of the lungs. In deep sleep, at the body's metabolic nadir, the scalenes become the primary muscles of inspiration because very small movements are needed. During waking, they primarily stabilize the sides of the neck. If they are also overloaded with the burden of daytime chest breathing—hard work for these small muscles— trigger points and significant pain can develop.

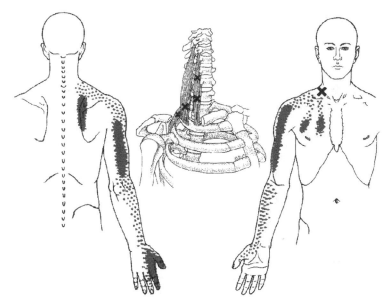

Fig. 13-5. The scalenes have a wide-ranging pain pattern and are very sensitive to breathing dysfunction.

For their small size, the scalenes have a wide-ranging pain pattern that can confuse practitioners who aren't well versed in trigger point therapy. The scalenes are one of the primary causes of pain felt between the shoulder blades, rendering it useless to spend a lot of energy doing massage on the muscles in that area. They also can cause strong anterior shoulder pain, high chest pain, and radial side pain extending down the forearm to the hand. These symptoms are likely to be diagnosed in any number of misguided ways, including cervical radiculopathy, tendinitis, carpal tunnel syndrome, bursitis, rotator cuff tears, and much more. They can cause thoracic outlet syndrome by hoisting the first rib up too close to the clavicle, forming a vice that compresses the structures of the thoracic nerve outlet.

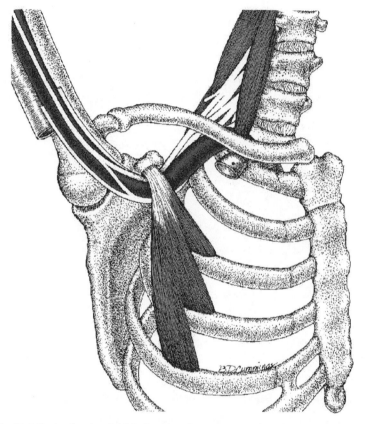

Fig. 13-6. Pectoralis minor in high chest breathers can cause thoracic outlet symptoms by entrapping nerves and blood vessels.

Pectoralis minor is a "canary in the coal mine" muscle that is vulnerable to overuse during chest breathing. It attaches the top of the scapula to the rib cage, so it's capable of elevating the rib cage to increase lung volume. It also crosses over the nerves and blood vessels of the thoracic outlet before they enter the arm, and if it develops taut fibers, it can produce true thoracic outlet syndrome.

Pectoralis minor is also one of the important muscles behind protracted, rounded shoulder posture. It will pull the scapula anteriorly if it adaptively shortens because it attaches to the coracoid process at the top of the scapula. This muscle is a primary antagonist of the low trapezius, which keeps the scapula positioned down on the back, just as the middle trapezius fibers are antagonistic to middle serratus anterior fibers. Both of these trapezius groups tend to get long and functionally weak because they are overpowered by their breathing-sensitive antagonists. I can't overemphasize the role of these relationships in establishing and maintaining some of the most severe and pervasive pain conditions that we see.

BREATHING, STRESS, AND SELF-PROTECTION

We've seen an epidemic of shoulder pain and frozen shoulder diagnoses in the last few years. Many factors have converged to set this up. We are under assault in our modern world with new levels of stress, particularly in the last few years, with the onslaught of social media, a global pandemic, social and political conflict, climate change—and our omnipresent mobile devices constantly bringing it all into our awareness. Even in the absence of acute events, the human response to stress tends to revert to the primitive protective reflex. In his book *Somatics*, Thomas Hanna uses the term "Red Light Reflex" to describe this neuromuscular response to stress, also known as the withdrawal response, escape response, or startle reflex. This response is in our primitive brain and occurs automatically if, for example, we hear a sudden loud sound. The shoulders lift and round forward, the head drops forward to protect the front of the neck, the abdomen tightens and flexes the lumbar spine, and breathing moves into the upper chest because the abdomen is compressed and the diaphragm cannot easily move the viscera out of the way. Interestingly, drug addicts instinctively revert to this posture during withdrawal.

Chest breathing is intimately connected to the self-protective response, as is engagement of the muscles that elevate and protract the scapula: the high trapezius, levator scapulae, high and mid serratus anterior, clavicular branch of pectoralis major, and pectoralis minor. It's not a coincidence that individuals who routinely chest breathe tend to carry higher levels of stress and anxiety; anxiety clinics teach diaphragmatic breathing as one of the first strategies for reducing anxiety and fear, a practice that has been shown to improve effect and attention and reduce cortisol levels in response to stress.[47] These are the same muscles that tend to engage and overpower the scapular retractors and depressors, leaving the scapula in a rounded, protracted position—a potent recipe for shoulder pain. Once it begins, the habit of abdominal engagement and shallow chest breathing creates a downward spiral that is hard to undo.

Chest breathing can be reversed, but it must be done slowly. Bodywork can be an important first step because a chronic chest breather is likely to have trigger points in their torso. Patients who have been chest breathing for several years will often find it very difficult to engage the diaphragm, and it might actually be painful for them to allow the belly to expand due to trigger points and taut fibers in the obliques and rectus abdominis, creating a negative incentive for change. Many of these patients have actually lost the ability to engage the diaphragm and allow it to push the viscera out, which requires firing the diaphragm while relaxing the abdominal wall muscles.

---

47 Xiao Ma, et al., "The Effect of Diaphragmatic Breathing on Attention, Negative Affect and Stress in Healthy Adults," *Frontiers in Psychology* 8, June 6, 2017, https://doi.org/10.3389/fpsyg.2017.00874.

In addition, there tends to be a collapse at the costal margin, where the ribs meet the abdominal wall. The obliques become shortened and pull on the ribs, making it difficult to stand up straight. And the rectus abdominis refers a band of back pain that can cross directly over the QL and the spinal erectors. All of the muscles in the low back are then subject to satellite referral, harden, and develop taut fibers.

The pain caused by chronic chest breathing is an example of both antagonist referral and reciprocal referral. Rectus abdominis refers into the spinal erectors, which are already overloaded from having to restrain the forward collapse of the thorax, and they then develop taut fibers, which make them resistant to shortening. If the person tries to manually correct their posture, their erectors will contract on shortening and cramp. The iliocostalis group (the most lateral spinal erector) refers through the abdomen to the front, which returns the favor to the rectus abdominis. This circular referral from front to back to front can powerfully perpetuate the collapsed posture once it is in place.

Many forces converge to develop and maintain this state of collapse and chronic pain. Women in particular report learning at a young age to keep their bellies hard and breathe with their chest, and this concern about physical appearance can embed physical and emotional trauma in the most vulnerable part of the body. I once worked with a woman who had grown up in eastern Europe. She was concerned about the appearance of her shoulders, which looked narrow and protracted, and she carried a lot of discomfort in her shoulders and neck. I did a bodywork session in which I corrected her scapular positioning and collapsed posture and assessed her for hyperpronation. When she looked at herself in the mirror, tears rolled down her face. She told me she had never seen herself with an open, erect posture and wide shoulders. When she was young, her parents had sent her to a "posture camp," which was shaming and traumatizing. Ironically, the early trauma produced the opposite effect, causing her to wear her negative self-esteem in her collapsed posture.

EMOTIONAL RELEASE AND FUNCTIONAL BREATHING

When we assist the body in releasing these self-protective patterns, many patients experience an emotional release. Trauma is held physically as well as emotionally, and bodywork often interacts with emotional change. Through manual therapy work we can temporarily give the client the experience of being open, unprotected, and upright, which presents a new reality and possibility to their central nervous system.

Nowhere do these issues coincide more directly than in the abdomen and breathing. Just being able to open the collapsed abdomen and chest to the world and taking diaphragmatic breaths without pain can be a powerful signal for emotional change. It can even modify blood chemistry by increasing oxygenation.

Once we've made it physically easier for the patient to breathe from the abdomen, the patient will need to confront the barriers of habit, body memory, old embedded self-protective strategies, and stored trauma to change their breathing patterns. Some will need to reacquaint themselves with their diaphragm and relearn how to use it to initiate breath. Changing the habit of breathing from the chest requires a great deal of patience and awareness, but it can be very rewarding.

One approach I recommend calls for the patient to lay supine, placing one hand on their belly and another touching their neck, particularly the SCMs and scalenes. Have them initiate a long, slow breath. The hand on the belly should move up as the diaphragm displaces the viscera. Notice if the neck muscles engage; the patient should aim to initiate breath without using the neck muscles at all. Have them do this exercise several times a day until they have changed their breathing habits. When first learning to engage the diaphragm, they might find themselves just pushing the belly out rather than using the diaphragm to do so indirectly, but this won't produce any in breath. The client must rediscover conscious control over the diaphragm by observing what causes inhalation to occur. Resting a weighted pillow on the belly can also provide some helpful proprioceptive feedback.

Once there is comfort with the basic procedure of diaphragmatic breathing, awareness must be brought to the breath as often as possible. While the new habit might get lost during times of stress, any reduction in the load on the chest and neck muscles will begin to pay off with less anxiety, pain, and tension. It can be done.

If you just do bodywork to help a patient with their pain issues but never deal with the perpetuating factors, the body will drift back into the same adaptations. Real change must happen at the level of the CNS, but our work with the musculoskeletal system can dramatically facilitate lasting change.

"Over the past five years, I've provided dozens of clients with shoe corrections that have tremendously helped their functioning in everyday life and helped keep their pain away. But my own experience with shoe correction is my favorite. I was in class with Chuck, learning about hyperpronation, and I decided to ask a question to get a better sense for how to identify it in a client. He began to answer me but then paused when he looked down at my feet. 'You are a hyperpronator,' he said. What he refrained from saying at that moment, perhaps as to keep from freaking me out, was that I have one of the more extreme cases of hyperpronation. And, in fact, I had been diagnosed with flat feet years earlier, a common hyperpronator's misdiagnosis considering I have perfectly healthy arches. That day changed my life. Chuck assessed me, fit me for insoles, and on our lunch break, I called my mom to explain to her why the two of us had such 'bad' knees and how I was going to keep myself from having to get them replaced like she did. Within days I realized my low back and shoulder pain had subsided. Then I eventually got some proper shoes that could also provide me the ankle support I needed, and stuffed with my tailored insoles, I was able to run down the block for the first time in my life without feeling like I was going to twist my ankle. I haven't gone without insoles since, and I have become the CTB poster child for hyperpronation. And more importantly, my shoulder pain from forward head posture has completely subsided, and I no longer have low back pain. Such a simple fix to pain I had been getting on and off for years."

—Zoë Verdin, CTB advanced practitioner and CTBI school administrator

CHAPTER 14

CTB and Movement: Yoga, Fitness, and Athletics

Many of our students have successfully applied CTB concepts to their existing practice in various modalities of coached movement, including yoga, Pilates, Gyrotonic, personal training, athletic training, dance, and other practices. These activities all challenge muscle and joint movements and tend to reveal issues with muscle dysfunction due to trigger points, which often limit a practitioner's ability to pursue their exercise or art. Depending on the modality, the trainer or instructor may choose to use some of our manual therapy techniques with their clients to help them understand and eliminate their pain, or they may model self-care techniques on themselves and then have the client do the same techniques.

When muscles are freed from trigger point dysfunction, they are stronger and can move with more fluidity and without pain, resulting in better balance, athletic performance, and resistance to injury. Allowing a client to continue their practice without having to take a break or avoid painful movements has significant benefits in terms of momentum, consistency, and maintaining a positive, enthusiastic attitude.

This chapter introduces some ideas on how to employ CTB concepts in your teaching or personal practice. The focus is primarily on yoga—because of my own personal experience—but you can apply the analysis and techniques to any form of movement or exercise.

Using CTB Principles in Yoga Practice

As a yoga practitioner myself for many years, I know that it's a powerful discipline that can be very helpful but can also be problematic if misunderstood or used too aggressively. A significant percentage of my students have come from the yoga world, and many of them are yoga teachers who feel lost when it comes to helping students who approach them about pain. Many people are drawn to yoga classes because they believe that yoga will help alleviate their pain through stretching and strengthening the body. However, most yoga teacher training programs fail to give teachers useful tools for therapeutic intervention or quality functional anatomy and trigger point training that focuses on the actual muscle effects of the poses.

While yoga teacher training programs vary tremendously among styles, anatomy training in these programs generally tends to be minimal. Many yoga teacher training programs only briefly cover the static location of muscles with the body in anatomical position, which gives trainees little useful or memorable information for a profession that is centered on joint movements. This reality is unfortunate because many people try yoga to seek relief from chronic pain.

Yoga asana—the physical poses—challenge, stretch, and shorten muscles, which can bring out significant pain and discomfort. A CTB-trained instructor with thorough training in functional anatomy and trigger point theory—including how muscles function dynamically in movement—can use this evidence to assess the true source of a student's pain and provide hands-on treatment. The instructor can also coach the student through self-care techniques that allow the student to move more fully into the asana, accruing its benefits without being blocked by a wall of pain.

I've made it a priority to reach and welcome yoga teachers and practitioners into my training programs. I believe that yoga teachers have a tremendous opportunity to lift people out of the dreadful cycle of injury-based thinking, painkillers, and surgery fostered by the pain industry and truly create change in millions of peoples' lives—but only if they are armed with the right analytical tools. The spiritual learning and self-awareness brought by a focused yoga practice have enormous benefits in terms of providing comfort, security, and central downregulation. Adding the muscle and trigger point knowledge amplifies the ability of yoga to provide tangible, physical relief.

Yoga teachers who study CTB learn extremely effective interventions that they can do with bodywork or self-care to help their students move into challenging new poses. The CTB approach can quickly unravel the compensations via informed manual interventions, an understanding of functional relationships, and attention paid to perpetuating factors. Practitioners can supercharge a practice like the Ashtanga Primary Series, helping them move more quickly into the essential strengthening and balancing elements of the practice without fighting through pain. Discomfort is fine, as long as it's not extreme. Severe pain upregulates the CNS and works against progress.

Just as I did with the Thai massage repertoire, my team and I have analyzed common yoga poses for muscular effects and likely pain symptoms. If a muscle has trigger points, then engagement, extreme lengthening, or shortening tends to produce pain in different ways. When a student has pain in a pose, most teachers will have them modify to avoid the pain, but this approach never challenges the dysfunction and misses an opportunity for long-term relief.

CTB training gives the teacher the knowledge they need to analyze the muscular effects of poses, as well as interpret symptoms that arise via direct and satellite pain referral from the affected muscles. A trained CTB therapist understands which muscles are complaining and blocking poses, and they can provide suitable interventions so the student can progress. They can then apply an appropriate selection of CTB treatment approaches, using neurological hacks to turn off the pain response instead of avoiding poses that hurt. They can do this through hands-on work in class or in private sessions or via teaching their students self-care techniques and constructive modifications rather than simply avoiding pain. Even just understanding the muscular origins of pain in yoga poses and teaching students to use contract/relax can be very effective.

A thorough knowledge of trigger point theory and functional anatomy is essential for analyzing muscular effects and understanding where pain originates. Our course offerings include a thorough Functional Anatomy class, which is quite popular with yoga teachers. The trigger point characteristics of each muscle are a core part of the course. We offer a CTB Fundamentals class as well, and these two provide all the background needed to bring CTB work into a yoga or movement class. I've taught my Functional Anatomy class in many yoga studios, and inevitably, we have an enjoyable time analyzing and correcting pain that students and teachers feel in specific poses. I enjoy this work because it can help people quickly, and it models how the teacher can contribute actively to their students' healing.

We are constantly adding to our yoga-specific offerings. For more info, please use the QR code later in this chapter or go to the following link: coachingthebody.com/yoga/.

MY OWN YOGA JOURNEY

I began practicing hatha yoga on my own in my teens, teaching myself from books. At that time, I was mostly interested in the spiritual and philosophical aspects of yoga, and I was naturally flexible, so the poses came easily to me. I didn't yet understand that my flexibility was, in some ways, a curse. I regularly had back spasms that would cripple me for a few days, and only much later did I realize that this was due to instability in my lumbar spine, imbalance in the deep spinal stabilization muscles, chronic hyperlordosis (excessive curve in the lower back), the influences of hyperpronation, and a leg length discrepancy. None of the yoga I was doing properly addressed those issues. I practiced the hatha poses statically, with no movement or transitions between them.

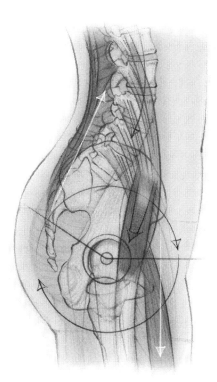

Fig. 14-1. Excessive lumbar curve and anterior pelvic tilt can be strongly perpetuated by trigger points and short, taut fibers in the lumbar spinal erectors and hip flexors.

In fact, as I continued my practice and sought in-person instruction over the years, I found that other teachers and styles of yoga emphasize keeping extension in the lumbar spine, even during a forward fold, so the lumbar never goes into flexion. In my own attempt to do so, I perpetuated my postural imbalance and placed all of the burden of flexion into the hips and lengthening the hamstrings. My body drifted into a constant state of hyperlordosis. My lumbar spinal erectors and QL muscles adaptively shortened and developed trigger points, and my hip flexors had shortened as well. For anyone, being in a persistent state of lumbar extension is unhealthy and is accompanied by a constant anterior pelvic tilt. This misalignment is difficult to reverse. I had been correcting my leg length discrepancy and hyperpronation for a few years, and that did dramatically reduce my back pain episodes, but I still had unbalanced strength and tension in my lumbar extensors and flexors. I had become an example of how the body over-stabilizes hypermobility over time, but my muscles had not compensated in a balanced way.

Later in life, after I had already started working with trigger point therapy and developing the CTB system, I began practicing in the ashtanga style. Ashtanga uses consistent sequences based on held poses along with choreographed movements—vinyasa—between the poses and a focus on breath and attention. Practicing the same sequence on a regular basis allows the practitioner to observe the ways in which their body changes with the practice.

Ashtanga students first learn a sequence called the Primary Series.[48] The Primary Series begins with surya namaskar (sun salutation), which focuses on spinal flexion and extension to develop balanced strength and flexibility in the spine. Not surprisingly, the ashtanga practice was very painful for me at first. Whenever

48 Ashtanga has a reputation for causing injuries by pushing too hard, and that is something that must be carefully managed by the instructor, and more importantly, by the practitioner.

I did a forward fold, I would feel severe pain in my lumbar spine from attempting to lengthen muscles that had shortened over many years. The first few months were tough, and I had to go very slowly. After many weeks, the pain began to ease, and I felt that my lumbar spine could move into flexion and extension rather than being locked in hyperlordotic extension.[49]

APPLYING CTB TO SPECIFIC ASANA

The next section includes a sample breakdown of a few common yoga poses as well as how to apply CTB analysis protocols. These principles can be applied to any pose. In order to understand any other yoga asana, we must analyze the muscle effects that are happening at each joint as it departs from anatomical position. When analyzing a pose not included here, first look at the joint actions, which tell you what muscles are lengthening or shortening. Then make a list of the muscles being affected, and examine their direct and satellite referral patterns to see what might be contributing to the pain.

One additional note: If you are having difficulty in any pose, I recommend using the contract/relax technique. If you find that going farther into a pose brings out symptoms, come out of the pose a bit and find a way to reverse the action against resistance. For example, if you're having trouble in triangle pose as you drop your torso toward the mat, hold on to your leg or foot with your lower hand, press into the floor with your front foot and try to lift and rotate up against the resistance. This will engage the muscle groups that may be resisting the stretch. Hold your breath for five seconds, and as you exhale, slowly drop farther into the stretch,

---

49 At that time, I had yet to discover the benefits of therapeutic vibration or design our therapeutic vibration tool, the Muscle Liberator. If I had, I would have used it to distract the nervous system, soften the spinal erectors and greatly accelerate my ability to move into lumbar flexion.

ideally using vibration on the areas where you feel discomfort. You can do two or three cycles of contract/relax and should be able to see a lot of improvement. At some point, as you increase stretch, that muscle's antagonists will increasingly shorten and begin to cause a different type of pain. You would then go into a treatment cycle on those muscles before trying to go any farther.[50]

Many of these interventions can be done by the practitioner on their own body, although sometimes having an instructor or therapist assisting is easier logistically.

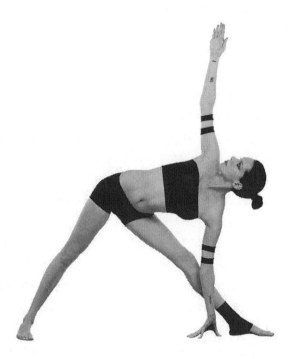

Fig. 14-2. Trikonasana (triangle pose). Nina Mel, Yoga Teacher, Creative Commons Attribution 3.0 Unported.

---

50 The ashtanga practice has a certain amount of contract/relax and a great deal of active stretching built into it, which is very helpful and intelligent, but in some cases, the order of events isn't ideal for someone who is already in a lot of pain. In my case, even with the contract/relax that occurred by engaging the spinal erectors prior to the forward fold, it was just terribly painful in the beginning.

MARICHYASANA A

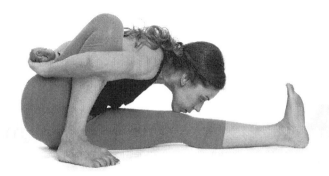

Fig. 14-3. Marichyasana A pose.

Marichyasana is a challenging pose series with four variations that occur in the middle of the Ashtanga Primary Series practice. The practitioner sits on the floor, one leg straight in front of the body or bent and the other bent with the heel near the hips. The main muscle effect in all variations is extreme hip flexion on one side, accompanied by other challenges depending on the variation. I will use marichyasana A as an example here. In this variation, the practitioner binds one arm around the bent leg, clasping the hands together behind the back. This bind pushes the torso forward, increasing hip flexion as well as flexion in the lumbar spine. The straight leg introduces a hamstring stretch. In other variations, both legs are bent. Typical complaints in this pose might include hip and groin pain, low back pain, and radiating pain in the medial or posterior leg. The binding of the arms may produce shoulder pain.

Important Muscle Effects
In this pose, the torso moves over the bent leg, potentially introducing a significant degree of hip flexion in relation to the position

of the pelvis. This produces a strong stretch on hip extensors such as adductor magnus and gluteus maximus. Despite its name, adductor magnus is more than a simple adductor; it's very involved in extending the leg at the hip, antagonistic to the TFL. With this much hip flexion, the extensor fibers of adductor magnus are in extreme stretch. With any deep stretch, some muscles inevitably shorten just as thoroughly, which can produce even greater challenges than the stretch component. In this case, all hip flexors are shortened, particularly iliacus, psoas major and minor, pectineus, and TFL, and the adductor longus is shortened and pressed up against the pelvis. The lumbar spinal erectors are placed on stretch, and the bind forces flexion throughout the spine. Consequently, the abdominal wall muscles and hip flexors will be shortened. The arms are in medial rotation, which might challenge infraspinatus. The more longitudinal QL fibers—bilateral lumbar extensors—will be placed under stretch.

Likely Challenges

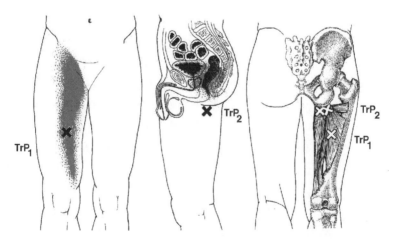

Fig. 14-4. Adductor magnus referral. Adductor magnus undergoes strong stretch in all versions of marichyasana.

Practitioners often report pinching in the groin on the bent knee side, and this can thoroughly limit their ability to move into the pose. Few people understand the concept of shortening dysfunction, which is what causes this difficulty. When a muscle contracts on short, you could feel cramping in the muscle itself, as well as its referral pattern. The iliacus—a strong one-joint hip flexor—is placed on extreme shortening in this pose, and its referral can go into the anterior thigh and groin. The iliopsoas, which includes iliacus, also can throw referral over the stretching lumbar spinal erectors, compromising them with satellite referral. This is a case of referral over a muscle's antagonist, which can set up a particularly potent opportunity for dysfunction.

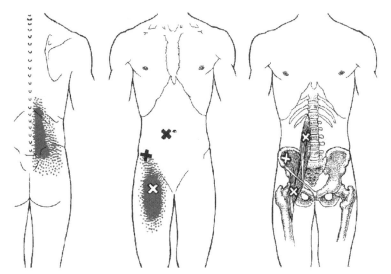

Fig. 14-5. The iliacus and psoas referrals can cause serious discomfort in marichyasana because of contraction on short. Used under license Photo 32499451 / Marichyasana © Guruxox | Dreamstime.com.

The adductors can also produce severe problems in this pose. Adductor longus is shortened, and its referral also lands in the groin and can cause satellite referral into the pectineus. Further, adductor magnus, whose extensor fibers are being placed under deep stretch, throws satellite referral directly over adductor longus. TFL, which is directly antagonistic to adductor magnus, can cause pain wrapping into the anterior thigh. Pectineus causes mostly local groin referral and is a satellite of adductor longus.

From a stretch perspective, you will feel the adductor magnus stretch in the muscle itself as well as its referral more medial on the thigh. The hamstrings may refer pain throughout the posterior thigh and behind the knee. The QLs under stretch may cause a wide-ranging referral into the glutes, abdomen, groin, and lateral leg.

Therapeutic Interventions

The most powerful intervention to ease deeper movement into this pose would involve therapeutic vibration from the Muscle Liberator. The basic approach involves taking the adductor magnus off extreme stretch, then using vibration on the muscle, finding areas of tenderness. You should also treat a client's adductor longus and TFL with vibration.

To contract/relax when in the pose, have your client drive the foot of their bent leg down into the mat and press the leg in toward their body's centerline with an inhale. Have them hold for five or more seconds, and on exhale, have them move further into the pose without binding as you use vibration on their adductor magnus, adductor longus, and TFL. Let them come out of the pose, and let the spinal erectors soften as you use vibration over them and the QLs. This can be done as self-care as long as the client can reach around to their back. Have the client arch their back into extension, then hold their breath for five seconds. On exhale, have them come into some lumbar flexion as you use vibration again over the low back. Ask the client to try the pose again. Any remaining pinch in the groin can be lessened by pressing your fingers into the area where they feel the most pain and using repeated contract/relax on the adductor magnus.

You can treat the adductor longus, adductor magnus, TFL, and low back with balls, cane, or vibration, but the client needs to come out of the pose temporarily. In the absence of any tools, the teacher can guide the student through contract/relax on the important agonists and antagonists in the pose, or they can use our bodywork protocols for the muscles if the setting is a private session or group in which that is appropriate. For a simple adjustment, the student can also contract the adductor magnus by driving the foot down into the mat, followed by moving into the pose with the teacher providing firm fingertip feedback into the shortening hip flexors and the adductor magnus.

The iliacus and hamstrings can also cause complications in this post. The iliacus can be problematic on shortening, so an additional intervention is for the teacher or practitioner to hook their fingers over the anterior part of the iliac spine, pressing against the inside of the pelvis. This compresses the fringe of the iliacus and can be held as you move into the pose.

If the hamstring stretch response is dominant and strong pain is felt behind the leg and knee, have the student bend their straight leg somewhat and engage the hamstrings for several seconds as they hold an inhale. On exhale, have them move deeper into the pose. As the pose deepens and the hamstrings let go, other muscles may begin to cause more noticeable discomfort, particularly on the shortening side.

DOWNWARD-FACING DOG

Downward-facing dog (or adho mukha svanasana) is a common pose in virtually all yoga styles. In spite of being considered a beginning pose, it presents many challenges for beginners.

Important Muscle Effects

Downward-facing dog requires 180 degrees of shoulder flexion to fully enter the pose. Some hypermobile individuals allow the arm to go past 180 degrees of flexion, but core engagement and lifting the torso out of extreme hyperflexion at the shoulders is far more beneficial than letting the chest collapse passively toward the floor.[51]

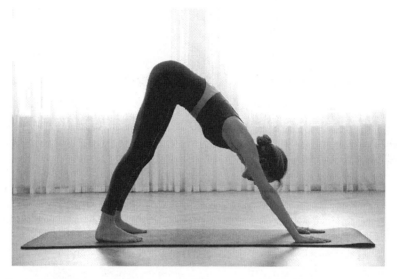

Fig. 14-6. The downward-facing dog pose challenges dorsiflexion, hip flexion, and scapular rotation. Used under license Photo 208762963 / Downward Facing Dog© Chernetskaya | Dreamstime.com.

The arm and scapula will naturally medially rotate in the pose, and the scapulas tend to adduct toward the spine, producing narrow shoulders. The practitioner should work to keep the shoulder blades wide and externally rotate the arms. To achieve full arm flexion, the scapula must be able to rotate upward, requiring proper range and coordination in the trapezius, rhomboids,

---

51 Hypermobile individuals need to emphasize strength-based practice, because hypermobile joints are somewhat unstable, and over time the body is likely to recruit trigger points in muscles to stabilize.

and serratus anterior. Rotation will often be limited in anyone with shoulder pain.

Hip flexion ideally is 90 degrees or more and will be strongly limited by insufficient hamstring length. Ankle dorsiflexion will depend upon the hip flexion angle, and if the practitioner must bend their knees because of short hamstrings, this will increase dorsiflexion angle. The gastrocnemius is placed on strong stretch if the knee is straight and heels are on the ground.

Likely Challenges

Shoulder and mid-back pain. This pose will readily bring out limitations in scapular positioning and motion. Arm flexion and abduction require that the scapula fully rotate. For every 30 degrees of total arm motion, the scapula should contribute approximately a third of the motion (10 degrees). One hundred eighty degrees of total arm motion in this pose would demand 60 degrees of scapular rotation.

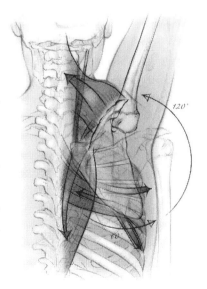

However, many people have limited scapular rotation and will likely present with a protracted, rounded shoulder when at rest. In these cases, serratus anterior fibers will have adaptively shortened and developed trigger points, pulling the scapula into protraction. The posterior fibers that pull against the serratus, namely mid/low trapezius and rhomboids, also tend to develop trigger points

Fig. 14-7. Full arm flexion requires full scapular and glenohumeral rotation.

and can cause mid-back, shoulder, head, and neck pain. The student is likely to have their shoulders elevated, floating up to their ears. In these cases, it's not generally useful or helpful to remind them to drop their shoulders because they simply can't manage to achieve enough arm flexion without elevating the scapula.

Satellite referral can wreak havoc in the shoulder. When the serratus is challenged, it will also refer into the low trapezius, setting up the entire low to high trapezius satellite pattern, perhaps even resulting in headaches. Additionally, other shoulder muscles will likely become dysfunctional, and many of them refer down the arm to the hand and wrist, as does the serratus anterior.[52]

Another challenge is pain in the front of the ankle. The considerable amount of dorsiflexion in downward-facing dog will shorten the tibialis anterior muscle (in the shin) and possibly cause painful contraction on the short. Tibialis anterior referral includes the front of the shin, front of the ankle, and the big toe line on the top of the foot. The ankle might also be very limited in dorsiflexion, as tibialis anterior disturbance generally accompanies issues in the soleus, which limits dorsiflexion. In this

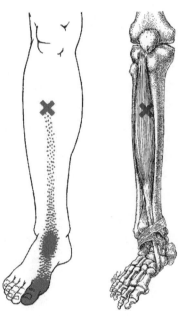

Fig. 14-8. Tibialis anterior referral. Anterior ankle pain is a common result.

52 Wrist pain may have little or nothing to do with the wrist itself. If the student is very limited in wrist extension, they might be painfully challenging the forearm flexors, many of which refer pain to the wrist. Conversely, forearm extensors might be contracting on short, causing pain on the dorsal side of the forearm and wrist. The subscapularis is also a strong wrist pain source.

case, even a mild amount of dorsiflexion may cause painful tibialis anterior contraction on short.

If the knees are straight in this pose, dorsiflexion will also lengthen the gastrocnemius (a calf muscle), which can refer pain into the Achilles tendon area and the plantar surface of the foot, as does the soleus. The posterior calf can easily be satellites of the hamstrings and posterior gluteus minimus referral, so those muscles must be included in treatment.

In general, glute issues are common in yoga teachers and practitioners. There is a high incidence of hypermobility and hyperpronation in this population, and the glutes try to stabilize the ankle against collapse, resulting in radiating sciatic referral in the hips, lateral, and posterior legs, including the hamstrings.[53]

Therapeutic Interventions

Shoulders: Even a single Core Upper Body Protocol treatment can significantly improve scapular rotation. An experienced, efficient practitioner can perform the scapular positioning protocol in fifteen to twenty minutes. Alternatively, the student can use a self-care routine as described in our Treat Your Own Shoulder Pain course. For a quick on-the-spot adjustment in the pose, have the student intentionally round and elevate their shoulders as they press the hands into the ground, holding with an inhale for five or more seconds. On exhale, ask them to let their chest sink toward the mat, pulling the scapula down and onto the back. This will influence many of the fibers that limit scapular motion.

---

53 For a long time, I was puzzled at how many of my yoga clients had so-called hamstring pain, when their hamstrings were much longer than what is considered normal. Treating the hamstrings never worked. Once I fully understood the origins and importance of gluteal satellite referral, it all made sense, and I could treat the source of their pain, rather than the location of it.

Lower leg: The CTB Core Lower Body Protocol features tibialis anterior/soleus treatment in the very beginning. Even twenty minutes of this work can transform ankle mobility and tibialis anterior trigger points. A quick contract/relax can be done by pressing into the mat with the ball of the foot, elevating the heel, holding with breath for five seconds, and then letting the heel drop closer to the mat. If pain is felt in the front, however, this will shorten the tibialis anterior even more and could make that pain worse. The downside to increasing range is that some muscles are likely to incur further shortening and express more pain, which is why it's always best to work both sides of the joint. The shortening pain in front of the ankle may feel like a damaged joint, but as we know, that pain is likely the result of trigger point referral.

FOLDED LEG POSES (LOTUS POSE, EASY POSE, HALF LOTUS)

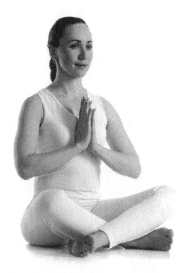

Fig. 14-9. Easy pose requires less external hip rotation than lotus pose. Used under license Photo 70879227 © Fizkes | Dreamstime.com.

The seated postures with legs folded appear at the end of the Ashtanga Primary Series and are common in most yoga styles and many meditation practices. Some individuals may struggle with these poses due to limitations in their gluteal fibers, lower back, and adductors.

Important Muscle Effects

All seated crossed-leg poses require a degree of external rotation at the hip, which can be the primary challenge for many people.

Padmasana, or lotus pose, requires the most extreme external rotation, as the ankle of one leg is raised up over the thigh of the other.

The common understanding of the function of gluteus medius and minimus fibers is that the anterior fibers medially rotate the femur, and the posterior fibers laterally rotate, which is true in anatomical position (lying on the back, arms at the sides, with palms facing up). However, Travell and Simons note that once the femur reaches 90 degrees of hip flexion, all gluteal fibers become medial rotators.[54] As the knee drops toward the mat in the crossed leg seated poses, the leg moves into increasing external rotation. For this reason, stretching in the glutes limits the folded leg poses to varying degrees.

Likely Challenges

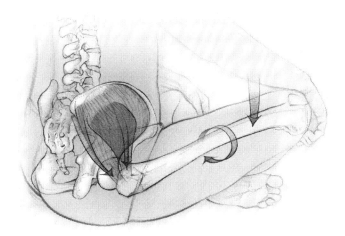

Fig. 14-10. Gluteal stretch produced by external rotation of the femur in folded leg poses.

---

54 Travell and Simons, *Myofascial Pain and Dysfunction: The Trigger Point Manual Vol. 2., The Lower Extremities*, 153.

When stretched, gluteus medius fibers will refer pain to the sacrum, low back, and glutes, while gluteus minimus refers a sciatic pain pattern radiating down the leg along with gluteal referral. Medial or lateral knee pain may occur due to satellite referral into the quads as well as compression in the knee joint if the student tries to force the pose. These symptoms are all likely to show up in the pose itself because the weight of the legs naturally carries them into more external rotation, stretching the gluteal fibers (anterior in particular). It's tempting to blame the adductors if the pose is uncomfortable, but the motion of dropping the knees to the floor doesn't significantly change adduction in this position.

Students with very tight gluteal fibers might be extremely uncomfortable even in a mild pose such as easy pose (sukhasana, sitting cross-legged without stacking the shins). Because gluteus medius is the most common muscle that causes low back referral, low back pain often occurs in people who have tight hips and find it difficult to sit cross-legged in any of these poses.

Therapeutic Interventions

A yoga instructor with solid CTB training can observe a student in a pose and assess the compensations that occur in the student's muscles. In some cases, a simple contract/relax with proper adjustment feedback can make a huge difference. A student who struggles with sitting cross-legged will likely need some focused treatment on the glutes, QL, TFL, and adductors. Our crossed-leg forward fold resolving stretch in the Core Lower Body Protocol is an assisted version of this posture.

In my CTB workshops for yoga, I often work with students who are extremely uncomfortable sitting. When I apply CTB techniques to them, we can quickly unlock their limitations. In a workshop on yoga anatomy, I assisted a woman who had experienced discomfort for years in the seated poses. I briefly worked with her glutes and then did a series of contract/relaxes in the seated forward fold assisted stretch. On the third repetition, she was able to fold forward fully over her crossed legs. She looked up at her yoga instructor and began crying.

Using CTB Principles in Training and Athletics

When working with particularly active people such as athletes, we need to understand that pain issues develop in muscles that are perpetually challenged and to look at misconceptions that many athletes and personal trainers have about pain.

INCORPORATING CTB SELF-CARE INTO CORRECTIVE EXERCISE

Any exercise or movement practice quickly reveals issues as muscles are asked to work, shorten, and stretch. Whenever you push muscles to develop more strength, there is some risk of acute overload, which can lead to trigger points. If severe, pain may interfere with the exercise. When we catch these developments before further neurological compensations occur, they are relatively easy to clear. In CTB corrective exercise, we use these symptoms as an assessment tool and combine self-care or bodywork with strength work.

If someone develops pain that interferes with their training, the CTB protocols provide a guide for analysis. Rather than simply modifying the exercise routine to avoid the pain, we teach our students to use it as an opportunity to rehabilitate the muscles and quickly return to resistance training. When we deal with issues as they arise, the CNS can integrate the new level of functionality, and the training itself becomes a therapeutic experience that can reduce pain overall via positive neuroplastic change. Post-exercise soreness can be reduced or eliminated, as some soreness is due to acute overload and trigger points.

Example: Therapeutic Serratus Anterior Resistance Training

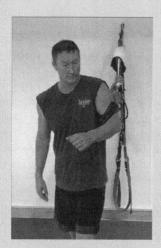

Fig. 14-11. Engaging serratus anterior by projecting the shoulder forward against resistance from a band.

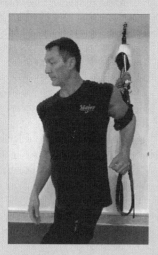

Fig. 14-12. The strap carries the shoulder back into retraction, for a serratus stretch.

At CTBI, we employ bodyweight exercise using a device called the Mighty Body Band. This device is similar to a TRX in some ways, with the addition of bungee cables for variable resistance as well as a waist strap. Basic resistance bands can be used for this purpose as well. We generally try to set up the exercise so that contract/relax can be performed seamlessly at any time. Active contraction against resistance will encourage the muscle to stay at a shorter resting length, and in the case of serratus anterior, the muscle often is already too short, dominating its antagonists and pulling the scapula into protraction. Additionally, any resistance work runs a risk of introducing new trigger points and taut fibers due to temporary acute overload. Particularly with serratus, we want to keep the muscle strong but long, balanced in its relationship with the trapezius and rhomboids.

Toward this goal, we intersperse some resistance work with stretching, but we do the stretch in the form of contract/relax, ideally with vibration on the stretch phase. You can do this with a TRX, a homemade strap, or pressing into the wall. To work serratus anterior, project your entire shoulder forward into the resistance

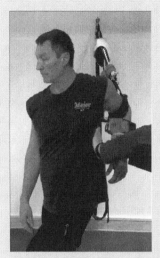

Fig. 14-13. Doug Ringwald applying therapeutic vibration on serratus during the relax phase.

for a few seconds. You can do five or ten repetitions and on the last rep of the set, hold resistance with an inhale and after five seconds or so, let the strap carry your shoulder back, turning away to increase the stretch if you wish.

You might feel some referred pain on the stretch, having just worked the muscle prior to contract/relax. I recommend using vibration on the stretch phase, just as we do in our self-care and bodywork protocols, as this will introduce a lot of neurological distraction to greatly facilitate the release of any new taut fibers that have developed. You can do this yourself or have someone else do it for you.

In this way, we can develop additional strength and push the muscle harder without throwing it into painful dysfunction. Particularly in the beginning of a training program, it's important to do strength training incrementally due to the fact that it's far easier to push untrained muscle fibers into overload, trigger points, and pain. Training in the manner described here clears new trigger points as they develop, and raises the threshold where the work crosses into counterproductive excess.

"Discovering CTB through my own pain experience was completely transformative. Years ago, I tore my medial meniscus in my right knee in a yoga class where I pushed myself into a yoga posture that I was not ready for. Being a runner for over a decade, I was used to pushing myself to reach my goals, but new to yoga. I brought the same competitive nature into my yoga practice and quickly learned my most valuable lesson. My strong desire and attachment to opening my hip quickly led to my knee taking the brunt of my force. I walked away with a swollen, injured knee that left me at a limit of 90 degrees of flexion with sharp pain and a significantly compromised gait for weeks. I was extremely discouraged as I was told surgery was the answer. Something inside of me cringed. My invincible nature quickly deflated, and I began my journey of what I call my true yoga practice. I turned down surgery and began to search for other ways to support my body's natural ability to heal. With surgery, I knew the incision of my joint capsule would be a guarantee for developing arthritis, according to the research I was reading. As I explored my options outside of the conventional medical model, I often pondered what did people do before the age of surgical intervention?! Humans have suffered from pain and injury as long as we've walked this planet...thousands and thousands of years. I was determined to find other ways to heal.

"Through acupuncture, myofascial release, mindfully practicing hot yoga, and massage, I increased my range of motion of knee flexion and began to walk again. I was relieved to know I avoided the conventional treatment of surgery and felt empowered by my body's ability to heal and repair. I gained about 90 percent of my function back but still struggled with certain movements and felt I was dancing around pain by avoiding certain movements as I felt my knee remained a bit unstable. I was mostly happy with my decision to avoid surgery but continued to be frustrated as I did not feel I had healed completely. A couple years later, I left a yoga class and felt my knee pain return even after being so cautious and mindful in my practice. I thought to myself that was it... I could hardly bear weight without sharp pain in my medial knee, and that I was headed to surgery after all. After talking with a few colleagues and learning that I did not suffer tissue damage but rather triggered a pain memory, I made a few phone calls.

This led me to a CTB Practitioner, Laura. I decided this was my last ditch effort, and I would be calling the surgeon later that day after seeing her. Something had to be done. I couldn't go on with this chronic instability, dysfunction, and pain. I was convinced it was a structural issue left over from the meniscus tear. Laura worked from my hip to my knee all the way down to my lower leg for over two hours, asking questions and following my answers around my body as she inquired about what I was feeling when she was working. I was amazed; it was like my body was telling her where to go and what to do, and she was listening... She used some tools that I was not familiar with at the time and was extremely detailed in her work. At the end of the session, I stood up, walked around the room, and I was flooded with emotion as I could walk freely with a steady gait, pain-free. Needless to say, I never called the surgeon.

"From that day forward, I have believed that we can heal from our pain and injuries completely, with skillful training, knowledge, and understanding of what the pain experience truly is and how our body functions as a whole, a complete and interconnected system, not the pieces and parts of the outdated reductionistic, injury-based perspective.

"Fast forward several years later... I have been fortunate to study in person with Chuck, Doug, and Zoe over the years and have built a full-time practice as a CTB Practitioner, RN, and Certified Yoga Therapist. I have recently opened my doors to my first Yoga Therapy & Wellness Studio, Lotus Care KC, in Gladstone, Missouri. I have anywhere between two to four clients every day, Monday through Friday, with great success in the protocols that Chuck has developed. I have treated frozen shoulders in a matter of two sessions, and I've helped many with chronic low back pain that surgery has failed. The combination of ancient wisdom with modern science has brought forth a new conversation and study in treating pain & dysfunction."

—Julianne Hutchcraft, RN, BSN,
C-IAYT yoga therapist and CTB practitioner

CHAPTER 15

Resources for Further Study

Neuroscientists have made amazing progress in understanding the underlying causes of pain. However, most therapists, medical personnel, and consumers still operate in an old, obsolete, injury-based model that just isn't accurate. They chase the potential pathology in the spine, joints, and connective tissue and ignore muscles as a potent source of nociception statistically most responsible for pain. The result has been a dismal record of failure, inappropriate use of pain medications, financial despair, ruined lives, addiction, and even death.

Neuroscience and trigger point therapy have largely remained separate disciplines, with little cross-pollination. While neuroscientists have mostly focused on central sensitization and neuroplastic change in their approach to chronic pain, networks of trigger points in muscles related by function and satellite referral operate silently, feeding the central nervous system with constant danger signals from the periphery. Trigger point therapy has been largely ignored because of its relatively inaccessible origins and the lack of a manual therapy system that applies trigger point principles with dynamic movement focused on supporting positive neuroplastic change in the CNS while also addressing peripheral dysfunction in muscles. Bodyworkers, having been taught ineffective trigger point techniques and an excessive focus on direct referral, have, to some degree, marginalized trigger point therapy as just another esoteric approach with a spotty track record.

My experience has been that trigger point practice is extremely effective when informed by an understanding of modern neuroscience, the true role of functional relationships and satellite referral, and improved techniques involving movement and distraction. Indeed, when used together, these concepts can fulfill the promise that excited Dr. Travell in her original research.

I was fortunate to have come to trigger point therapy with no preconceptions and a movement-oriented background in martial arts, yoga, and Thai massage. My prior career as a software researcher and programming language designer taught me the value of remaining curious and open, experimenting, and keeping what works. This was the ground out of which Coaching the Body emerged. After helping many people in my own practice, I'm gratified today that we have a good understanding of how to empower others to do this work through our training.

My purpose in writing this book has been to provide a ray of hope to the millions of people who suffer daily with chronic pain, to plant a seed with a broader network of therapists who can effectively apply these ideas, and to begin to change the broken system. I hope that I've given you something useful that will improve your own life in some way. It would not have been possible to cover our entire system in practical detail in a single book, so in this chapter, I'll leave you with some links for further study.

Becoming a Coaching the Body Practitioner

Coaching the Body Institute has been teaching practitioners since 2001. We build knowledge from the ground up that our students need of functional anatomy, trigger point theory, neuroscience, and bodywork. Our student base includes massage therapists, physical therapists, chiropractors, yoga teachers, trainers, and many others, including interested individuals with no background in the field. Our trainings offer NCBTMB-approved continuing education credits in massage, and credits are available for selected other professions as well.

Fig. 15-1. Classes landing page QR code.

We offer a multi-year virtual membership training that makes it easy to learn and apply CTB concepts from anywhere in the world, as well as individual virtual classes such as Functional Anatomy for Bodywork, Movement, and Yoga and CTB Fundamentals, both of which can be taken as first classes.

In-person study is available as well. However, in recent years we had to limit our offerings due to safety requirements during the pandemic. CTBI is headquartered in Evanston, Illinois, and our certified instructors also offer in-person coursework and mentoring in other parts of the country. For more information, scan the QR code in Figure 15-1 or visit coachingthebody.com/study/.

Resolving Your Own Pain with CTB Self-Care Courses

As we continue to expand our network of certified CTB practitioners, we're constantly deluged by requests for help from people in pain who have been unable to find relief via other methods. We've created online courses that teach anyone who is interested and motivated how to address the most common upper and lower body pain issues by applying CTB principles via our self-care techniques. These courses have been very successful, and practitioners also

Fig. 15-2. Self-care landing page QR code.

find them helpful as a resource library of self-care routines that they can give their clients. To learn more, scan the QR code in Figure 15-2 or visit coachingthebody.com/selfcare/.

Coaching the Body for Yoga

We at CTBI are very interested in helping yoga teachers understand the true sources of pain so they can assist their students via coaching, adjustments, and self-care. With millions of people attending yoga classes every day for help with their chronic pain, yoga teachers have a huge opportunity and also a responsibility to be a

Fig. 15-3
Yoga landing page
QR code.

guide for their students in stopping pain at the source. The CTB approach is highly compatible with yoga principles and techniques. We're expanding our coursework specifically to help yoga teachers understand the most common types of dysfunction that they will see in their students, along with a variety of interventions. For more information, follow the QR code in Figure 15-3 or visit coachingthebody.com/yoga/.

The PainHackers Directory

As our students become qualified to practice Coaching the Body successfully, they can be listed in our PainHackers Directory, which only lists students who have successfully completed portions of our training program. Visitors can search for qualified practitioners by ZIP code. Please scan the QR code in Figure 15-4 or visit painhackers.org.

Fig. 15-4
PainHackers
Directory QR code.

"My name is Rob Murray. After competing on the US National Skeleton Team towards the 2006 Winter Olympics, coaching, and eventually retiring from the sport, I wanted to delve into another modality of massage therapy and reconnect with my Thai heritage. Chuck was the only instructor across the country to return my dozen inquiries. I told him who I was and what I was interested in— the use of bodywork for performance enhancement and therapy for athletes (he understood immediately), and I enrolled into his first HandsFree Thai Massage course at his school in Evanston. After the first evening of class, I was sold on him, his instruction method, and his entire curriculum. We were instant friends; he has that kind of wise, calming presence. I implored him to teach me everything he knew and allow me to be his first teacher outside of Chicago. It has been an amazing journey in the resolution of pain for many of my clients, my own aches as a therapist, and the instruction of hundreds of my own students through Chuck Duff's program.

"I have been in sports medicine, massage therapy, and exercise science for nearly thirty years, and half of that time, I have worked closely with Chuck. This ever-evolving body of work yields efficient practices that allow me to work without excess strain on my own body, and because of this, I have helped many athletes and people through the knowledge I have gained: with hands-on instruction and teaching and my own work with and on clients.

"CTB is very well-suited for athletics. Many of my high school, recreational and professional athletes learn how to manage their bodies with the combination of workouts and recovery to which CTB is integrated and integral.

"For example, I have been treating an athlete for years in middle school as a swimmer, but in high school, he switched to running. As expected, the transition strained his muscles and hurt his performance. I have worked with him gradually and progressively increased his understanding and strength. We have created a base of knowledge on how to manage and treat his body, and with CTB in his senior year, we were able to accomplish a Cross-Country State Championship and athletic scholarship to an Ivy League school.

"Just recently, a client was complaining of a stiff lower back for weeks and after pursuing treatments with his doctors, getting physical therapy, imaging, and medications—having no better outcome or recourse, contacted me. After some careful questions, I was able to make an accurate assessment over the phone and resolve the complaint in a few minutes of CTB bodywork. For many issues, it's just that simple because the method is sound—tried and true—and for that understanding, I am forever grateful. I could not have asked for a better mentor, role model, or friend than Chuck Duff."

—Rob Murray ATC/L, LMT, CSCS, NSCA-CPT,
advanced CTB therapist and instructor, Orlando, Florida

ACKNOWLEDGMENTS

I count myself very fortunate every day to have my daughter, Rachel, in my life. She is a true friend, and her wisdom, humor, intelligence, and grace give me something to aspire to.

Love and gratitude to Spooky Trapasso, whose caring insight and support have sustained me through the challenges of realizing my work and who helped me build a world-class school from humble beginnings.

I would like to thank Doug Ringwald, the first student to certify as a master-level CTB therapist, for a rich and fruitful collaboration and friendship for the last several years of bringing these ideas to the world.

Much gratitude to Zoe for her hard work in organizing the school as we grew and for her care in shepherding hundreds of students through our programs.

I'm deeply thankful to Liz Hartley, whose love and friendship have been a stalwart anchor as I finished and published this book. As a multitalented teacher, artist, and acute observer of the world, she was instrumental in making the book better and keeping me intact to see it through.

Thank you to my student Will Baird, a talented therapist who was always willing to be a model for our video work and to help out in any way he could.

I am grateful beyond words to my coach, Leslie Sann, whose spiritual guidance and brilliant counsel have helped me to derive so much joy from my life and relationships, even when things are hard.

When I met Clair Davies, I was inspired by his story, a warm and eloquent former piano technician who became an expert trigger point therapist and author. His book and workshops were some of the key early influences that started me down this path.

Many thanks to Frank Scott, a talented acupuncturist who invited me to be a faculty member at Pacific College of Oriental Medicine, a potent proving ground where I continued to develop my work, learned a lot, and met some great people.

A note of appreciation to Dr. David Hanscom for his support, fascinating neuroscience discussions, and ongoing work in empowering people to understand and release chronic pain.

Dr. Lorimer Mosely has provided an entertaining and seminal body of neuroscientific work regarding the nature of pain. His ideas have been essential in my formulation of Coaching the Body.

This book would be nothing without the brilliant researchers who have been developing the science and system of trigger point therapy since the 1940s, without much attention or appreciation from mainstream medicine: Dr. Janet Travell, Dr. David Simons, Dr. Robert Gerwin, Dr. Jay Shah of NIH, Jan Dommerholt, and many more.

Big thanks to Mary Biancalana for her mentoring, friendship, guidance, caring, humor, and terrific Baggo tournaments. A talented trigger point therapist and teacher herself, Mary contributed in many important ways to my early development of the CTB system and invited me to be a frequent speaker at NAMTPT conferences.

Warm thanks to my advanced students, who have become pain experts and dear friends over the years: Rob Murray, Jill Duncan, Brent Doornbos, Julie Zuleger, Krista Matison, Donna, Heidi, and others. Special thanks to my advanced student Josh, who brainstormed the term Coaching the Body, and we all knew it was perfect.

I'm extremely appreciative of my content editor Abby and her monumental work in wrangling early versions of this book into something more coherent. Her efforts went well beyond the call of duty.

Special thanks to my amazing marketing team at NeedlesEye Media—Dorothy, I could not have gotten to where I am now without you. Gratitude to Jim for his amazing copywriting and leadership.

I was fortunate to come across the brilliant work of my illustrator, Juliet Percival—she brings excitement, art, and living beauty to the sometimes dry task of rendering anatomy.

Love and thanks to my dear friend Gary Bobroff, an author, Jungian therapist, teacher, and conference organizer who provided concrete encouragement and wisdom when I needed to just sit down and write. Participating in the Synchronicity conference was a fascinating experience that I will always fondly remember, along with our frequent talks during these trying times for the world.

Love and gratitude to my sister Rita and her husband Jack, and all of my nieces and nephews and their families who bring me love and joy and who I don't get to see often enough.

To Barbara Monier, whose friendship and experience as a talented and prolific author was an immense help in the early stages of this book.

My dear friend and music collaborator Doug Frohman has brought humor, companionship, wisdom, and joy to my life, and he enhances the world with his art. I always know he will be there when I need help.

Tim Anderson is a wonderful friend and brilliant artist who has always been a source of encouragement, laughter, and shared sushi at Kuni.

Jane Friedman and Mark Griffin offered some key advice and encouraged me to complete the project at a time when I needed some confidence. They come from a viewpoint of deep publishing expertise. And they make it fun.

The team at Scribe Media has been consistently impressive and a joy to work with, and it's clear that they care as much as I do about producing and delivering a top-quality book.

I have acquired key ideas along the journey from many more individuals, too numerous to mention here: therapists, anatomists, Rolfers, acupuncturists, trainers (a special thanks to Tommy Biancalana), and other teachers along the way.

Special thanks and respect to all of my Thai massage teachers and the people of Thailand, who developed a fascinating art that has provided a key foundation for my techniques.

BIBLIOGRAPHY

"50 Shades of Pain with Prof. Lorimer Moseley." Trust Me, I'm a Physiotherapist. Accessed April 17, 2021. https://trustmephysio-therapy.com/50-shades-of-pain-with-lorimer-moseley/.

American Physical Therapy Association. "7Staggering Statistics About America's Opioid Epidemic," May 9, 2016. https://www.choosept.com/resources/detail/7-staggering-statistics-about-america-s-opioid-epi.

Adler, Susan S., Dominiek Beckers, and Math Buck. *PNF in Practice: An Illustrated Guide*. Fourth fully revised edition. Berlin: Springer, 2014.

Baldry, Peter E. Acupuncture, *Trigger Points and Musculoskeletal Pain: A Scientific Approach to Acupuncture for Use by Doctors and Physiotherapists in the Diagnosis and Management of Myofascial Trigger Point Pain*. Edinburgh: Elsevier Churchill Livingstone, 2008.

Baliki, Marwan N., and A. Vania Apkarian. "Nociception Pain, Negative Moods and Behavior Selection." *Neuron* 87, no. 3 (August 5, 2015): 474–91. https://doi.org/10.1016/j.neuron.2015.06.005.

Bhattacharyya, Kalyan B. "The Stretch Reflex and the Contributions of C David Marsden." *Annals of Indian Academy of Neurology* 20, no. 1 (2017): 1–4. https://doi.org/10.4103/0972-2327.199906.

Borg-Stein, Joanne, and David G. Simons. "Myofascial Pain." *Archives of Physical Medicine and Rehabilitation* 83 (March 2002): S40–47. https://doi.org/10.1053/apmr.2002.32155.

Botter, Alberto, Taian M. Vieira, Tommaso Geri, and Silvestro Roatta. "The Peripheral Origin of Tap-Induced Muscle Contraction Revealed by Multi-Electrode Surface Electromyography in Human Vastus Medialis." *Scientific Reports* 10, no. 1 (February 10, 2020): 2256. https://doi.org/10.1038/s41598-020-59122-z.

Bron, Carel. *Myofascial Trigger Points in Shoulder Pain Prevalence, Diagnosis and Treatment.* S.l.; Nijmegen: s.n.]; Universiteitsbibliotheek Nijmegen [host, 2011. http://hdl.handle.net/2066/85865.

Bron, Carel, and Jan D. Dommerholt. "Etiology of Myofascial Trigger Points." *Current Pain and Headache Reports* 16, no. 5 (October 2012): 439–44. https://doi.org/10.1007/s11916-012-0289-4.

Bron, Carel, et al. "The Prevalence of Shoulder Girdle Muscles with Myofascial Trigger Points in Patients with Shoulder Pain." *BMC Musculoskeletal Disorders* 12, no. 1. Accessed April 7, 2021. https://www.academia.edu/14078807/High_prevalence_of_shoulder_girdle_muscles_with_myofascial_trigger_points_in_patients_with_shoulder_pain.

Bron, Carel, et al. "Treatment of Myofascial Trigger Points in Patients with Chronic Shoulder Pain: A Randomized, Controlled Trial." *BMC Medicine* 9, no. 1. Accessed May 18, 2021. https://www.academia.edu/14078806/Treatment_of_myofascial_trigger_points_in_patients_with_chronic_shoulder_pain_a_randomized_controlled_trial.

Burke, Robert E. "Sir Charles Sherrington's the Integrative Action of the Nervous System: A Centenary Appreciation." *Brain: A Journal of Neurology* 130, no. Pt 4 (April 2007): 887–94. https://doi.org/10.1093/brain/awm022.

Chaitow, Leon. "Might Trigger Points Sometimes Be Useful?" Leon Chaitow. Accessed September 18, 2020. https://leonchaitow.com/2009/04/14/might-trigger-points-sometimes-be-useful/.

Chaitow, Leon. *Muscle Energy Techniques (Advanced Soft Tissue Techniques)* (London: Pearson Professional Limited, 1996).

Chen, Jun. "History of Pain Theories." *Neuroscience Bulletin* 27, no. 5 (September 29, 2011). https://doi.org/10.1007/s12264-011-0139-0.

"Chronic Pain and the Brain." Physiopedia. Accessed April 23, 2021. https://www.physio-pedia.com/Chronic_Pain_and_the_Brain.

Chu, Jennifer, I. Schwartz, and S. Schwartz. "Chronic Refractory Myofascial Pain: Characteristics of Patients Who Self-Select Long-Term Management with Electrical Twitch-Obtaining Intramuscular Stimulation." *International Journal of Physical*

Chu, Jennifer, Frans Bruyninckx, and Duncan V. Neuhauser. "Chronic Refractory Myofascial Pain and Denervation Supersensitivity as Global Public Health Disease." *BMJ Case Reports.* Accessed June 10, 2021. https://www.academia.edu/26391176/Chronic_refractory_myofascial_pain_and_denervation_supersensitivity_as_global_public_health_disease.

Cramer, Gregory D., Susan A. Darby, and Gregory D. Cramer. *Clinical Anatomy of the Spine, Spinal Cord, and ANS.* 3rd ed. St. Louis, Mo: Elsevier, 2014.

Dahlhamer, James. "Prevalence of Chronic Pain and High-Impact Chronic Pain Among Adults—United States, 2016." *Morbidity and Mortality Weekly Report* 67 (2018). https://doi.org/10.15585/mmwr.mm6736a2.

Davies, Clair, Amber Davies, and David G. Simons. *The Trigger Point Therapy Workbook: Your Self-Treatment Guide for Pain Relief.* 2nd Edition. Oakland, CA: New Harbinger Publications, 2004.

DeLaune, Valerie. *Trigger Point Therapy for Repetitive Strain Injury: Your Self-Treatment Workbook for Elbow, Lower Arm, Wrist and Hand Pain.* A New Harbinger Self-Help Workbook. Oakland, CA: New Harbinger Publications, 2012.

Doidge, Norman. *The Brain That Changes Itself: Stories of Personal Triumph from the Frontiers of Brain Science.* 1st edition. Penguin Books, 2007.

Doidge, Norman. *The Brain's Way of Healing: Remarkable Discoveries and Recoveries from the Frontiers of Neuroplasticity.* Updated edition. New York, New York: Penguin Books, 2016.

Dommerholt, Jan, Carel Bron, and Jo Franssen. "Myofascial Trigger Points: An Evidence-Informed Review." *Journal of Manual & Manipulative Therapy* 14 (October 1, 2006): 203–21. https://doi.org/10.1179/106698106790819991.

Dommerholt, Jan, and Robert D. Gerwin. "A Critical Evaluation of Quintner et al: Missing the Point." *Journal of Bodywork and Movement Therapies* 19, no. 2 (April 2015): 193–204. https://doi. org/10.1016/j.jbmt.2015.01.009.

Dommerholt, Jan, Rob Grieve, Michelle Layton, and Todd Hooks. "An Evidence-Informed Review of the Current Myofascial Pain Literature—January 2015." *Journal of Bodywork and Movement Therapies* 19, no. 1 (January 2015): 126–37. https://doi.org /10.1016/j.jbmt.2014.11.006.

Donnelly, Joseph M, César Fernández-de-Las-Peñas, Michelle Finnegan, and Jennifer L. Freeman. *Travell, Simons & Simons' Myofascial Pain and Dysfunction: The Trigger Point Manual.* 3rd edition. Philadelphia: LWW, 2018.

Duff, Charles. "Designing an Efficient Language." *BYTE Magazine* Vol. 11:8 (August 1987): 211–24, https://vintageapple.org/byte/ pdf/198608_Byte_Magazine_Vol_11-08_Object-Oriented_ Languages.pdf.

Duff, Charles, and Iverson, Norman. "Forth Meets Smalltalk." *Journal of Forth Application and Research* 2, no. 3 (n.d.). https:// dl.forth.com:8443/jfar/vol2/no3/article1.pdf.

Fairclough, John, et al. "Is Iliotibial Band Syndrome Really a Friction Syndrome?" *Journal of Science and Medicine in Sport* 10, no. 2 (April 2007): 74–76; discussion 77–78. https://doi.org/10.1016/j. jsams.2006.05.017.

Fernández-Lao, Carolina, et al. "Myofascial Trigger Points in Neck and Shoulder Muscles and Widespread Pressure Pain

Hypersensitivtiy in Patients With Postmastectomy Pain: Evidence of Peripheral and Central Sensitization." *The Clinical Journal of Pain* 26, no. 9 (November 2010): 798–806. https://doi.org/10.1097/AJP.0b013e3181f18c36.

FRCA, Jane C. Ballantyne MD, Scott M. Fishman MD, and James P. Rathmell MD. Bonica's *Management of Pain*. 5th edition. Philadelphia: LWW, 2018.

Gerber, Naomi Lynn, Siddhartha Sikdar, Jen Hammond, and Jay Shah. "A Brief Overview and Update of Myofascial Pain Syndrome and Myofascial Trigger Points." *Journal of Spinal Research Foundation,* 6, no. 1 (2011): 10. https://www.semanticscholar.org/paper/A-Brief-Overview-and-Update-of-Myofascial-Pain-and-Gerber-D./2ae6c11f83ebd22e36a0487e2286b36e1644861a

Gevirtz, Richard. "The Muscle Spindle Trigger Point Model of Chronic Pain," *Biofeedback,* 34, no 2 (2006): 4. https://www.proquest.com/scholarly-journals/muscle-spindle-trigger-point-model-chronic-pain/docview/208145411/se-2.

Gladwell, Malcolm. *The Tipping Point: How Little Things Can Make a Big Difference*. Boston: Back Bay Books, 2002.

Gleiberman, Owen, and Owen Gleiberman. "'The Crime of the Century' Review: Alex Gibney's Shattering HBO Documentary Drills Deep into the Opioid Crisis." *Variety* (blog), May 3, 2021. https://variety.com/2021/film/reviews/the-crime-of-the-century-review-alex-gibney-hbo-the-opioid-crisis-1234963623/.

Hadizadeh, Monavar, et al. "Effects of Intramuscular Electrical Stimulation on Symptoms Following Trigger Points; A Controlled Pilot Study." *Journal of Modern Rehabilitation* 11, no. 1 (October 1, 2017): 3. https://doi.org/10.18869/nirp.jmr.11.1.31.

Hanna, Thomas. *Somatics: Reawakening The Mind's Control Of Movement, Flexibility, and Health*. Illustrated edition. Cambridge, MA: Da Capo Press, 2004.

Hanscom, David. *Back in Control: A Surgeon's Roadmap Out of Chronic Pain*, 2nd Edition. Vertus Press, 2016.

Hanscom, David. *Do You Really Need Spine Surgery?: Take Control with a Surgeon's Advice*. Vertus Press, 2019.

"History of Pain." The Pain Project. Accessed September 27, 2019. http://www.internationalreporting.org/pain/history-of-pain/

Hsieh, Yueh-Ling, et al. "Dry Needling to a Key Myofascial Trigger Point May Reduce the Irritability of Satellite MTrPs." *American Journal of Physical Medicine & Rehabilitation* 86, no. 5 (May 2007): 397–403. https://doi.org/10.1097/PHM.0b013e31804a554d.

Duff, Charles. "Ice Your Tissues, Freeze Your Issues—The Illusory Appeal of Icing." Coaching the Body, February 26, 2015. https://coachingthebody.com/ice-your-tissues-freeze-your-issues-the-downside-of-icing/.

Gendlin, Eugene T. "Plato's Dialectic," The Gendlin Online Library, 1966. http://previous.focusing.org/gendlin/docs/gol_2231.html.

Hales, Craig M. et al. "Prescription Drug Use Among Adults Aged 40–79 in the United States and Canada." Centers for Disease

Control and Prevention. August 8, 2019. https://www.cdc.gov/
nchs/products/databriefs/db347.htm.

"Introducing the Imprecision Hypothesis in Chronic
Pain." Rayner & Smale. Accessed April 24, 2021.
https://www.raynersmale.com/blog/2015/10/6/
introducing-the-imprecision-hypothesis-in-chronic-pain.

Irnich, Dominik. *Myofascial Trigger Points: Comprehensive
Diagnosis and Treatment.* Edinburgh: Churchill Livingstone/
Elsevier, 2013.

Itza, Fernando, et al. "Myofascial Pain Syndrome in the Pelvic
Floor: A Common Urological Condition." *Actas Urológicas
Españolas* (English Edition) 34, no. 4: 318–26. Accessed June 29,
2021. https://www.academia.edu/23932538/Myofascial_pain_syn-
drome_in_the_pelvic_floor_A_common_urological_condition?e-
mail_work_card=thumbnail.

"JCO Interview." *Journal of Clinical Orthodontics.* Accessed
September 26, 2019. https://www.jco-online.com/ar-
chive/1989/07/468-jco-interviews-janet-g-travell-md-on-myofas-
cial-pain/.

Jonckheere, Peter and Jan A J Pattyn. *Myofascial Muscle Chains.*
Newark: Trigger, 1998. 308.

Kellgren, J. H. "Referred Pains from Muscle." *British Medical
Journal* 1, no. 4023 (February 12, 1938): 325–27. https://www.
ncbi.nlm.nih.gov/pmc/articles/PMC2085707/.

Khan, Murad Ahmad, Fauzia Raza, and Iqbal Akhtar Khan. "Pain: History, Culture and Philosophy." *Acta Medico-Historica Adriatica*: 13, no. 1 (2015): 113–30. https://pubmed.ncbi.nlm.nih.gov/26203543/.

Kimura, Y., H.-Y. Ge, Y. Zhang, M. Kimura, H. Sumikura, and L. Arendt-Nielsen. "Evaluation of Sympathetic Vasoconstrictor Response Following Nociceptive Stimulation of Latent Myofascial Trigger Points in Humans." *Acta Physiologica* 196, no. 4 (August 2009): 411–17. https://doi.org/10.1111/j.1748-1716.2009.01960.x.

Konczak, Jürgen, and Giovanni Abbruzzese. "Focal Dystonia in Musicians: Linking Motor Symptoms to Somatosensory Dysfunction." *Frontiers in Human Neuroscience* 7 (June 25, 2013). https://doi.org/10.3389/fnhum.2013.00297.

Kostopoulos, Dimitrios, Arthur J. Nelson, Reuben S. Ingber, and Ralph W. Larkin. "Reduction of Spontaneous Electrical Activity and Pain Perception of Trigger Points in the Upper Trapezius Muscle through Trigger Point Compression and Passive Stretching." *Journal of Musculoskeletal Pain* 16, no. 4 (January 2008): 266–78. https://doi.org/10.1080/10582450802479594.

Kostopoulos, Dimitrios, and Konstantine Rizopoulos. *The Manual of Trigger Point and Myofascial Therapy*. Thorofare, N.J: Slack, 2001.

Lacomba, María Torres, et al. "Incidence of Myofascial Pain Syndrome in Breast Cancer Surgery: A Prospective Study." *The Clinical Journal of Pain* 26, no. 4: 320–25. Accessed May 22, 2021. https://www.academia.edu/17355712/Incidence_of_Myofascial_Pain_Syndrome_in_Breast_Cancer_Surgery_A_Prospective_Study.

Lari, Yeganeh, et al. "The Effect of the Combination of Dry Needling and MET on Latent Trigger Point Upper Trapezius in Females." *Manual Therapy* 21 (February 2016): 204–9. https://doi.org/10.1016/j.math.2015.08.004.

Lehman, Greg. "The Mechanical Case against Foam Rolling Your IT Band. It Can Not Lengthen and It Is Not Tight." Greg Lehman. March 17, 2012. http://www.greglehman.ca/blog/2012/03/17/stop-foam-rolling-your-it-band-it-can-not-lengthen-and-it-is-not-tight.

Lin, Ming-Ta, Hsin-Shui Chen, Li-Wei Chou, and Chang-Zern Hong. "Treatment of Attachment Trigger Points in the Gluteal Muscles to Cure Chronic Gluteal Pain: A Case Report." *Journal of Musculoskeletal Pain* 19, no. 1 (January 2011): 31–34. https://doi.org/10.3109/10582452.2010.538823.

Lucas, Karen R., Barbara I. Polus, and Peter A. Rich. "Latent Myofascial Trigger Points: Their Effects on Muscle Activation and Movement Efficiency." *Journal of Bodywork and Movement Therapies* 8, no. 3(2004): 160—66. https://www.academia.edu/6570575/Latent_myofascial_trigger_points_their_effects_on_muscle_activation_and_movement_efficiency.

Ma, Xiao, Zi-Qi Yue, et al. "The Effect of Diaphragmatic Breathing on Attention, Negative Affect and Stress in Healthy Adults." *Frontiers in Psychology* 8 (June 6, 2017). https://doi.org/10.3389/fpsyg.2017.00874.

Malanga, Gerard A., and Eduardo J. Cruz Colon. "Myofascial Low Back Pain: A Review." *Physical Medicine and Rehabilitation Clinics of North America* 21, no. 4 (November 2010): 711–24. https://doi.org/10.1016/j.pmr.2010.07.003.

McAtee, Robert E. *Facilitated Stretching*. 2nd ed. Champaign, IL: Human Kinetics, 1999.

McPartland, John M., and David G. Simons. "Myofascial Trigger Points: Translating Molecular Theory into Manual Therapy." *Journal of Manual & Manipulative Therapy* 14, no. 4 (October 2006): 232–39. https://doi.org/10.1179/106698106790819982.

Medicine & Rehabilitation 01, no. 04 (2013). https://doi.org/10.4172/2329-9096.1000134.

Meldrum, Marcia L. "Medical Biology: History of Pain Management." *ScienceWeek*, December 12, 2003. https://www.opioids.com/pain-management/history.html.

Menakam, P. T., and K. Kalaichandran. "Effect of Ischemic Compression Followed by Stretching on Myofascial Trigger Points" *International Journal of Scientific and Research Publications* 5, no. 1 (2015): 6.

Mills, Sarah E.E., Karen P. Nicolson, and Blair H. Smith. "Chronic Pain: A Review of Its Epidemiology and Associated Factors in Population-Based Studies." *British Journal of Anaesthesia* 123, no. 2 (August 2019): e273–83. https://doi.org/10.1016/j.bja.2019.03.023.

Moayedi, Massieh, and Karen D. Davis. "Theories of Pain: From Specificity to Gate Control." *Journal of Neurophysiology* 109, no. 1 (October 3, 2012): 5–12. https://doi.org/10.1152/jn.00457.2012.

Moseley, G. Lorimer, and Johan W. S. Vlaeyen. "Beyond Nociception." *PAIN* 156, no. 1 (January 2015): 35–38. https://www.academia.edu/14419850/Beyond_nociception.

Nahin, Richard L., Bryan Sayer, Barbara J. Stussman, and Termeh M. Feinberg. "Eighteen-Year Trends in the Prevalence of, and Health Care Use for, Noncancer Pain in the United States: Data from the Medical Expenditure Panel Survey." *The Journal of Pain: Official Journal of the American Pain Society* 20, no. 7 (July 2019): 796–809. https://doi.org/10.1016/j.jpain.2019.01.003.

Nath, Rahul K, and Sonya E Melcher. "Rapid Recovery of Serratus Anterior Muscle Function after Microneurolysis of Long Thoracic Nerve Injury." *Journal of Brachial Plexus and Peripheral Nerve Injury* 2 (February 9, 2007): 4. https://doi.org/10.1186/1749-7221-2-4.

Niddam, David M., Rai-Chi Chan, Si-Huei Lee, Tzu-Chen Yeh, and Jen-Chuen Hsieh. "Central Modulation of Pain Evoked From Myofascial Trigger Point." *The Clinical Journal of Pain* 23, no. 5: 440–48. Accessed September 1, 2021. https://www.academia.edu/4501721/Central_Modulation_of_Pain_Evoked_From_Myofascial_Trigger_Point.

Norrsell, Ulf, Stanley Finger, and Clara Lajonchere. "Cutaneous Sensory Spots and the 'Law of Specific Nerve Energies': History and Development of Ideas." *Brain Research Bulletin* 48, no. 5 (March 15, 1999): 457–65. https://doi.org/10.1016/S0361-9230(98)00067-7.

Oatis, Carol A. *Kinesiology: The Mechanics and Pathomechanics of Human Movement*. Third edition. Philadelphia: Wolters Kluwer, 2017.

"Opioid Overdose Crisis." National Institute on Drug Abuse, January 22, 2019. https://www.drugabuse.gov/drugs-abuse/opioids/opioid-overdose-crisis.

Page, Phillip, Clare C. Frank, and Robert Lardner. *Assessment and Treatment of Muscle Imbalance: The Janda Approach*. Champaign, IL: Human Kinetics, 2010.

"Pain Theories." Wikipedia, April 14, 2021. https://en.wikipedia. org/w/index.php?title=Pain_theories&oldid=1017738631.

Partanen, Juhani V., Tuula A. Ojala, and Jari P.A. Arokoski. "Myofascial Syndrome and Pain: A Neurophysiological Approach." *Pathophysiology* 17, no. 1 (February 2010): 19–28. https://doi. org/10.1016/j.pathophys.2009.05.001.

Phadke, V, PR Camargo, and PM Ludewig. "Scapular and Rotator Cuff Muscle Activity during Arm Elevation: A Review of Normal Function and Alterations with Shoulder Impingement." *Revista Brasileira de Fisioterapia* (Sao Carlos (Sao Paulo, Brazil)) 13, no. 1 (February 1, 2009): 1–9. https://doi.org/10.1590/S1413-35552009005000012.

"Prescription Drugs." Health Policy Institute. Accessed January 27, 2021. https://hpi.georgetown.edu/rxdrugs/.

Rajith, P., Sharay Agawal ,and L. Anand. "Revelation and Easy Management of Rhomboids Muscle Trigger Point as a Cause of Distressing Non-cardiac Chest Pain—A Case Series." *International Journal of Advanced Research* 4(2016): 72—80. https://www.academia. edu/28424063/REVELATION_AND_EASY_MANAGEMENT_OF_ RHOMBOIDS_MUSCLE_TRIGGER_POINT_AS_A_CAUSE_OF_ DISTRESSING_NON_CARDIAC_CHEST_PAIN_A_CASE_SERIES.

Reji, Rhea, Vasavi Krishnamurthy, and Mandavi Garud. "Myofascial Pain Dysfunction Syndrome: A Revisit." *IOSR Journal of Dental and Medical Sciences* 16, no. 01(2017): 13. https://

www.academia.edu/42107248/Myofascial_Pain_Dysfunction_
Syndrome_A_Revisit?email_work_card=view-paper.

Richler, Phihpp, and Eric Hebgrn. *Trigger Points and Muscle Chains in Osteopathy (Complementary Medicine)*. Stuttgart, Germany: Thieme, 2008. 242.

Rio, Ebonie, et al. "The Pain of Tendinopathy: Physiological or Pathophysiological?" *Sports Medicine*. December 28, 2013. https://doi.org/10.1007/s40279-013-0096-z.

Selby, Karen. "32 Chronic Pain Statistics to Help You Understand Your Health." Asbestos.com. Accessed April 6, 2021. https://www.asbestos.com/cancer/chronic-pain-statistics/.

Sergienko, Stanislav, and Leonid Kalichman. "Myofascial Origin of Shoulder Pain: A Literature Review." *Journal of Bodywork and Movement Therapies* 19, no. 1 (January 2015): 91–101. https://doi.org/10.1016/j.jbmt.2014.05.004.

Shah, Jay P. "New Frontiers in the Matrix of Neuro-Musculoskeletal Pain: Integrating Pain Mechanisms with Objective Physical Findings and Needling Strategies." (2012) 23.

Shah, Jay P., et al. "Biochemicals Associated With Pain and Inflammation Are Elevated in Sites Near to and Remote From Active Myofascial Trigger Points." *Archives of Physical Medicine and Rehabilitation* 89, no. 1 (January 2008): 16–23. https://doi.org/10.1016/j.apmr.2007.10.018.

Shah, Jay P., and Elizabeth A. Gilliams. "Uncovering the Biochemical Milieu of Myofascial Trigger Points Using in Vivo Microdialysis: An

Application of Muscle Pain Concepts to Myofascial Pain Syndrome." *Journal of Bodywork and Movement Therapies* 12, no. 4 (October 2008): 371–84. https://doi.org/10.1016/j.jbmt.2008.06.006.

Shah, Jay P., et al. "Myofascial Trigger Points Then and Now: A Historical and Scientific Perspective." *PM & R: The Journal of Injury, Function, and Rehabilitation* 7, no. 7 (July 2015): 746–61. https://doi.org/10.1016/j.pmrj.2015.01.024.

Sherrington, Charles Scott. *The Integrative Action of the Nervous System*. New Haven Yale University Press, 1920. http://archive.org/details/integrativeactio00sheruoft.

Sikdar, Siddhartha, et al. "Understanding the Vascular Environment of Myofascial Trigger Points Using Ultrasonic Imaging and Computational Modeling." *2010 Annual International Conference of the IEEE Engineering in Medicine and Biology*. September 4, 2010. https://www.academia.edu/675636/Understanding_the_vascular_environment_of_myofascial_trigger_points_using_ultrasonic_imaging_and_computational_modeling.

Sikdar, Siddhartha, et al. "Novel Applications of Ultrasound Technology to Visualize and Characterize Myofascial Trigger Points and Surrounding Soft Tissue." *Archives of Physical Medicine and Rehabilitation* 90, no. 11 (November 2009): 1829–38. https://doi.org/10.1016/j.apmr.2009.04.015.

Simons, David G., and Jan Dommerholt. "Myofascial Pain Syndromes—Trigger Points." *Journal of Musculoskeletal Pain* 13, no. 4 (January 2005): 39–48. https://doi.org/10.1300/J094v13n04_08.

Smith, Rusty, Cynthia Nyquist-Battie, Mark Clark, and Julie Rains. "Anatomical Characteristics of the Upper Serratus Anterior: Cadaver Dissection." *Journal of Orthopaedic and Sports Physical Therapy*, 33(8) (2003): 449–54. https://www.researchgate.net/publication/10571942_Anatomical_Characteristics_of_the_Upper_Serratus_Anterior_Cadaver_Dissection.

Souza, Juliana Barcellos de, et al. "Prevalence of Chronic Pain, Treatments, Perception, and Interference on Life Activities: Brazilian Population-Based Survey." *Pain Research and Management*. 2017. https://doi.org/10.1155/2017/4643830.

Starlanyl, Devin. "Fibromyalgia and Chronic Myofascial Pain: Keys to Diagnosis and Treatment." 2003, 8.

Sulżycki, Paul Valdemar. "The Brain Behind Myofascial Trigger Points," n.d., 76.

Travell, J., and N. H. Bigelow. "Referred Somatic Pain Does Not Follow a Simple 'Segmental Patter.'" *Federation Proceedings 5*, no. 1 Pt 2 (1946): 106.

Travell, Janet. *Office Hours: Day and Night. Ex-Library edition.* The World Publishing Company, 1969.

Travell, Janet G., and David G. Simons. *Myofascial Pain and Dysfunction: The Trigger Point Manual; Vol. 2., The Lower Extremities.* Baltimore: LWW, 1992.

Travell, Janet, Seymour Rinzler, and Myron Herman. "Pain And Disability of the Shoulder And Arm: Treatment by Intramuscular Infiltration with Procaine Hydrochloride." *Journal of the American*

Medical Association 120, no. 6 (October 10, 1942): 417–22. https://doi.org/10.1001/jama.1942.02830410005002.

Travell, Janet, and David Simons. *Myofascial Pain and Dysfunction, Vol. 1: The Trigger Point Manual, The Upper Extremities. 1st Edition.* Baltimore: Williams & Wilkins, 1982.

Treaster, D., William S. Marras, D. Burr, James E. Sheedy, and D. Hart. "Myofascial Trigger Point Development from Visual and Postural Stressors during Computer Work." *Journal of Electromyography and Kinesiology: Official Journal of the International Society of Electrophysiological Kinesiology* 16, no. 2 (April 2006): 115–24. https://doi.org/10.1016/j.jelekin.2005.06.016.

Twilley, Nicola. "The Neuroscience of Pain." *The New Yorker*. June 25, 2018. https://www.newyorker.com/magazine/2018/07/02/the-neuroscience-of-pain.

Ullrich, Peter. "Failed Back Surgery Syndrome (FBSS): What It Is and How to Avoid Pain after Surgery." *Spine-health*. Accessed September 11, 2021. https://www.spine-health.com/treatment/back-surgery/failed-back-surgery-syndrome-fbss-what-it-and-how-avoid-pain-after-surgery.

"Upper-Crossed Syndrome." *Physiopedia*. Accessed February 2, 2021. https://www.physio-pedia.com/Upper-Crossed_Syndrome.

Wahrman, Anna and Whitney Akers. "Chronic Pain: How We're Losing the Battle," *Healthline*. November 9, 2017. https://www.healthline.com/health-news/america-is-losing-the-war-on-chronic-pain.

Wang, Chao, et al. "Spatial Pain Propagation Over Time Following Painful Glutamate Activation of Latent Myofascial Trigger Points in Humans." *The Journal of Pain* 13, no. 6(2012): 537–45. https://www.academia.edu/16808430/Spatial_Pain_Propagation_Over_Time_Following_Painful_Glutamate_Activation_of_Latent_Myofascial_Trigger_Points_in_Humans.

Wheeless' *Textbook of Orthopaedics.* "Section 4, Chapter 2: Epidemiology and Use of Opioids in Back Pain," August 31, 2020. https://www.wheelessonline.com/issls/section-4-chapter-2-epidemiology-and-use-of-opioids-in-back-pain/.

Wilson, Virginia P. "Janet G. Travell, MD." *Texas Heart Institute Journal* 30, no. 1 (2003): 8–12. https://www.ncbi.nlm.nih.gov/pmc/articles/PMC152828/.

Zelaya, Carla E. et al. "Chronic Pain and High-impact Chronic Pain among US Adults, 2019." Centers for Disease Control and Prevention." November 2020, https://www.cdc.gov/nchs/products/databriefs/db390.htm.

Zugasti, Aitor Martın-Pintado, et al. "Effects of Spray and Stretch on Postneedling Soreness and Sensitivity After Dry Needling of a Latent Myofascial Trigger Point." *Archives of Physical Medicine and Rehabilitation,* June 10, 2014, https://pubmed.ncbi.nlm.nih.gov/24928191/#:~:text=Conclusions%3A%20The%20spray%20and%20stretch,are%20related%20to%20postneedling%20pain.